Heart Failure

Guest Editor

PRAKASH C. DEEDWANIA, MD, FACC, FACP, FASH, FAHA

MEDICAL CLINICS OF NORTH AMERICA

www.medical.theclinics.com

September 2012 • Volume 96 • Number 5

SAUNDERS an imprint of ELSEVIER, Inc.

W.B. SAUNDERS COMPANY
A Division of Elsevier Inc.

1600 John F. Kennedy Boulevard • Suite 1800 • Philadelphia, Pennsylvania 19103-2899

http://www.theclinics.com

MEDICAL CLINICS OF NORTH AMERICA Volume 96, Number 5
September 2012 ISSN 0025-7125, ISBN-13: 978-1-4557-3892-2

Editor: Pamela Hetherington

Medical Clinics of North America (ISSN 0025-7125) is published bimonthly by Elsevier Inc., 360 Park Avenue South, New York, NY 10010-1710. Months of issue are January, March, May, July, September, and November. Periodicals postage paid at New York, NY, and additional mailing offices. Subscription prices are USD 232 per year for US individuals, USD 424 per year for US institutions, USD 117 per year for US students, USD 295 per year for Canadian individuals, USD 551 per year for Canadian institutions, USD 184 per year for Canadian students, USD 358 per year for international individuals, USD 551 per year for international institutions and USD 184 per year for international students. To receive student/resident rate, orders must be accompanied by name of affiliated institution, date of term, and the *signature* of program/residency coordinator on institution letterhead. Orders will be billed at individual rate until proof of status is received. Foreign air speed delivery is included in all *Clinics* subscription prices. All prices are subject to change without notice. **POSTMASTER:** Send address changes to *Medical Clinics of North America*, Elsevier Health Sciences Division, Subscription Customer Service, 3251 Riverport Lane, Maryland Heights, MO 63043. **Customer Service: Telephone: 1-800-654-2452** (U.S. and Canada); **1-314-447-8871** (outside U.S. and Canada). **Fax: 1-314-447-8029. E-mail: journalscustomerservice-usa@elsevier.com** (for print support); **journalsonlinesupport-usa@ elsevier.com** (for online support).

Reprints. For copies of 100 or more of articles in this publication, please contact the Commercial Reprints Department, Elsevier Inc., 360 Park Avenue South, New York, NY 10010-1710. Tel.: 212-633-3812; Fax: 212-462-1935; E-mail: reprints@elsevier.com.

Medical Clinics of North America is also published in Spanish by McGraw-Hill Interamericana Editores S. A., P.O. Box 5-237, 06500 Mexico, D.F., Mexico.

Medical Clinics of North America is covered in *MEDLINE/PubMed (Index Medicus), Current Contents, ASCA, Excerpta Medica, Science Citation Index, and ISI/BIOMED.*

Printed in the United States of America.

MEDICAL CLINICS OF NORTH AMERICA

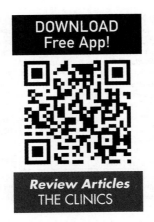

GOAL STATEMENT

The goal of *Medical Clinics of North America* is to keep practicing physicians up to date with current clinical practice by providing timely articles reviewing the state of the art in patient care.

ACCREDITATION

The *Medical Clinics of North America* is planned and implemented in accordance with the Essential Areas and Policies of the Accreditation Council for Continuing Medical Education (ACCME) through the joint sponsorship of the University of Virginia School of Medicine and Elsevier. The University of Virginia School of Medicine is accredited by the ACCME to provide continuing medical education for physicians.

The University of Virginia School of Medicine designates this enduring material activity for a maximum of 15 *AMA PRA Category 1 Credit*(s)™ for each issue, 90 credits per year. Physicians should only claim credit commensurate with the extent of their participation in the activity.

The American Medical Association has determined that physicians not licensed in the US who participate in this CME enduring material activity are eligible for a maximum of 15 *AMA PRA Category 1 Credit*(s)™ for each issue, 90 credits per year.

Credit can be earned by reading the text material, taking the CME examination online at http://www.theclinics.com/home/cme, and completing the evaluation. After taking the test, you will be required to review any and all incorrect answers. Following completion of the test and evaluation, your credit will be awarded and you may print your certificate.

FACULTY DISCLOSURE/CONFLICT OF INTEREST

The University of Virginia School of Medicine, as an ACCME accredited provider, endorses and strives to comply with the Accreditation Council for Continuing Medical Education (ACCME) Standards of Commercial Support, Commonwealth of Virginia statutes, University of Virginia policies and procedures, and associated federal and private regulations and guidelines on the need for disclosure and monitoring of proprietary and financial interests that may affect the scientific integrity and balance of content delivered in continuing medical education activities under our auspices.

The University of Virginia School of Medicine requires that all CME activities accredited through this institution be developed independently and be scientifically rigorous, balanced and objective in the presentation/discussion of its content, theories and practices.

All authors/editors participating in an accredited CME activity are expected to disclose to the readers relevant financial relationships with commercial entities occurring within the past 12 months (such as grants or research support, employee, consultant, stock holder, member of speakers bureau, etc.). The University of Virginia School of Medicine will employ appropriate mechanisms to resolve potential conflicts of interest to maintain the standards of fair and balanced education to the reader. Questions about specific strategies can be directed to the Office of Continuing Medical Education, University of Virginia School of Medicine, Charlottesville, Virginia.

The faculty and staff of the University of Virginia Office of Continuing Medical Education have no financial affiliations to disclose.

The authors/editors listed below have identified no professional or financial affiliations for themselves or their spouse/partner:

Jagroop Basraon, DO; Javed Butler, MD, MPH; Enrique Carbajal, MD; Susan Cheng, MD; Punam Chowdhury, MD; Rajiv Choudhary, MD, MPH; Robert T. Cole, MD; Vasiliki Georgiopoulou, MD; Gregory Giamouzis, MD; John Groarke, MBBChBAO, MSc; Pamela Hetherington, (Acquisitions Editor); Andreas Kalogeropoulos, MD, PhD; Joel A. Lardizabal, MD; Amirali Masoumi, MD; Patrick McCann, MD; Javid Moslehi, MD; Vijaiganesh Nagarajan, MD, MRCP; Shradha Rathi, MD; Dan Tong, MD, PhD; Filippos Triposkiadis, MD; and Andrew Wolf, MD (Test Author).

The authors/editors listed below identified the following professional or financial affiliations for themselves or their spouse/partner:

Kanu Chatterjee, MB, FRCP(Lond), FRCP (Edin), FCCP, MACP is a consultant for Gilead.

Prakash C. Deedwania, MD (Guest Editor) is a consultant and is on the Speakers' Bureau for Forest Pharmaceuticals and Pfizer, Inc., is on the Advisory Board for Pfizer, Inc., and is on the Speakers' Bureau for Takeda.

Paul J. Hauptman, MD is on the Advisory Board for Otsuka America Pharmaceutical Inc and BioControl Medical Inc, is on the Speakers' Bureau for Otsuka America Pharmaceutical Inc and Medcape Journal, is the Associate Editor for the American Heart Association, receives research support from Celladon Corp, National Heart, and is the Clinical Trials Investigator in the Heart Failure Network for the Lung and Blood Institute.

Jay Khambhati, BA, BS receives research support from the American Cancer Society.

Alan Maisel, MD receives research support from Alere, Abbott, and Critical Diagnostics; is a consultant for Alere; is on the Speakers' Bureau for Critical Diagnostics and Brahms; and is on the Advisory Board for and owns stock in Critical Diagnostics.

W.H. Wilson Tang, MD is a consultant for Medtronic, Inc. and St. Jude Medical, is receives research support from Abbott Laboratories.

Disclosure of Discussion of Non-FDA Approved Uses for Pharmaceutical Products and/or Medical Devices.

The University of Virginia School of Medicine, as an ACCME provider, requires that all faculty presenters identify and disclose any off-label uses for pharmaceutical and medical device products. The University of Virginia School of Medicine recommends that each physician fully review all the available data on new products or procedures prior to clinical use.

TO ENROLL

To enroll in the Medical Clinics of North America Continuing Medical Education program, call customer service at 1-800-654-2452 or visit us online at http://www.theclinics.com/home/cme. The CME program is available to subscribers for an additional fee of USD 228.

Contributors

GUEST EDITOR

PRAKASH C. DEEDWANIA, MD, FACC, FACP, FASH, FAHA
Professor of Medicine, Division of Cardiology, Fresno Medical Education Program, University of California-San Francisco, San Francisco, California; Chief of Cardiology, Cardiology Division, Veteran's Affairs Central California Health Care System, Fresno, California

AUTHORS

JAGROOP BASRAON, DO
Cardiology Fellow, University of California San Francisco, Fresno, California

JAVED BUTLER, MD, MPH
Division of Cardiology, Emory University, Atlanta, Georgia

ENRIQUE CARBAJAL, MD
Fresno Medical Education Program, Associate Clinical Professor of Medicine, Division of Cardiology, Department of Medicine, University of California San Francisco, San Francisco, California; VA Central California Health Care System, Fresno, California

KANU CHATTERJEE, MB, FRCP(Lond), FRCP (Edin), FCCP, FAHA, FACC, MACP
Clinical Professor of Medicine, The Carver College of Medicine, University of Iowa; Emeritus Professor of Medicine, University of California, San Francisco

SUSAN CHENG, MD
Division of Cardiovascular Medicine, Department of Medicine, Brigham and Women's Hospital, Boston, Massachusetts

RAJIV CHOUDHARY, MD, MPH
Capitol Health Medical Center, Trenton, New Jersey

PUNAM CHOWDHURY, MD
San Diego Veterans Affairs Medical Center; University of California San Diego, San Diego, California

ROBERT T. COLE, MD
Assistant Professor of Medicine, Division of Cardiology, Emory University, Atlanta, Georgia

PRAKASH C. DEEDWANIA, MD, FACC, FACP, FASH, FAHA
Fresno Medical Education Program, Professor of Medicine, Division of Cardiology, Department of Medicine, University of California-San Francisco, San Francisco, California; Chief of Cardiology, Cardiology Division, Veterans Affairs Central California System, VACCHS Medical Center, Fresno, California

VASILIKI GEORGIOPOULOU, MD
Division of Cardiology, Emory University, Atlanta, Georgia

GREGORY GIAMOUZIS, MD
Division of Cardiology, Larissa University Hospital, Larissa, Greece

JOHN GROARKE, MBBChBAO, MSc
Division of Cardiovascular Medicine, Department of Medicine, Brigham and Women's Hospital, Boston, Massachusetts

PAUL J. HAUPTMAN, MD
Professor of Medicine, Division of Cardiology, Saint Louis University School of Medicine, St Louis, Missouri

ANDREAS KALOGEROPOULOS, MD, PhD
Division of Cardiology, Emory University, Atlanta, Georgia

JAY KHAMBHATI, BA, BS
Division of Cardiovascular Medicine, Department of Medicine, Brigham and Women's Hospital, Boston, Massachusetts

JOEL A. LARDIZABAL, MD
Division of Cardiology, Department of Medicine, University of California-San Francisco (Fresno-MEP), Fresno, California

ALAN MAISEL, MD
San Diego Veterans Affairs Medical Center; University of California San Diego, San Diego, California

AMIRALI MASOUMI, MD
Division of Cardiology, Emory University, Atlanta, Georgia

PATRICK McCANN, MD
Division of Cardiology, Saint Louis University School of Medicine, St Louis, Missouri

JAVID MOSLEHI, MD
Division of Cardiovascular Medicine, Department of Medicine, Brigham and Women's Hospital; Division of Medical Oncology, Early Drug Development Center, Lance Armstrong Foundation, Dana-Farber Cancer Institute, Harvard Medical School, Boston, Massachusetts

VIJAIGANESH NAGARAJAN, MD, MRCP
Department of Hospital Medicine, Cleveland Clinic, Cleveland, Ohio

SHRADHA RATHI, MD
Cardiology Fellow, UCSF Fresno Cardiology, Fresno, California

DAN TONG, MD, PhD
Division of Cardiovascular Medicine, Department of Medicine, Brigham and Women's Hospital, Boston, Massachusetts

FILIPPOS TRIPOSKIADIS, MD
Division of Cardiology, Larissa University Hospital, Larissa, Greece

W.H. WILSON TANG, MD
Heart and Vascular Institute, Cleveland Clinic, Cleveland, Ohio

Contents

Heart failure (HF) remains a major growing public health problem in the United States. Despite extensive understanding of the mechanism at the molecular level and innovations in therapy, HF carries high morbidity and mortality rates, with frequent hospital admissions. In the Medicare population, HF is the leading cause for hospitalization, accounting for more than1 million admissions per year. The authors provide a review of the epidemiology and pathophysiology of HF.

Systolic and diastolic heart failure are the 2 most common clinical subsets of chronic heart failure. Left ventricular "Starling" function is depressed in patients with systolic heart failure. In systolic heart failure, left ventricular mass is increased, which can be measured by transthoracic echocardiography. Cardiac magnetic resonance imaging is a more precise technique to measure left ventricular mass. Neurohormonal activation is a major pathophysiologic mechanism for ventricular remodeling and progression of heart failure in systolic heart failure.

The activation of compensatory pathways and ongoing hemodynamic changes result in the release of biomarkers that can be monitored to chart disease progression and possibly target for therapy. We will review the biomarkers of heart failure that have been the focus of much discussion and research, including neurohormonal markers, particularly natriuretic peptides, cardiac injury markers, specifically troponins, inflammatory marker sST2, and matrix remodeling marker Galectin-3. In addition, we will discuss cardiorenal markers that have shown promise in improving risk stratification of patients with HF with worsening renal function, such as cystatin C, neutrophil gelatinase-associated lipocalin (NGAL), and kidneyinjury molecule-1 (KIM-1).

Heart failure (HF) is a major public health problem associated with increased morbidity and mortality. As the US life expectancy increases and the population ages, the overall prevalence of HF will continue to escalate. The increasing use of effective selective therapies such as neurohormonal blockade in the treatment of patients with HF has led to considerable improvement in the prognosis. During the past several decades, some studies have demonstrated the benefits of treatment; based on the evidence available from these studies, various national and international guidelines have specific recommendations for the evidence-based therapy with these drugs in patients with HF.

This review discusses the role of diuretics in heart failure by focusing on different classifications and mechanisms of action. Pharmacodynamic and pharmacokinetic properties of diuretics are elucidated. The predominant discussion highlights the use of loop diuretics, which are the most commonly used drugs in heart failure. Different methods of using this therapy in different settings along with a comprehensive review of the side-effect profile are highlighted. Special situations necessitating adjustment and the phenomenon of diuretic resistance are explained.

Inotropic therapy remains an option in the management of patients with advanced heart failure symptoms from systolic dysfunction who do not respond to conventional therapies. The decision to use this class is largely predicated on an accurate evaluation of the patient's fluid and perfusion status. Selection of the appropriate agent and dosing regimens requires an understanding of the underlying pathophysiology of heart failure and concomitant therapy. Most important, the goals of care should be stated clearly, given inherent risks associated with this class of drug.

Renal dysfunction is a common, important comorbidity in patients with both chronic and acute heart failure (HF). Chronic kidney disease and worsening renal function (WRF) are associated with worse outcomes, but our understanding of the complex bidirectional interactions between the heart and kidney remains poor. When addressing these interactions, one must consider the impact of intrinsic renal disease resulting from medical comorbidities on HF outcomes. WRF may result from any number of important processes. Understanding the role of each of these factors and their interplay are essential in understanding how to improve outcomes in patients with renal dysfunction and HF.

Multiple comorbidities are common in patients in heart failure. Some of them could contribute to the development of heart failure, whereas others may lead to disease progression and may be associated with poor prognosis. It is not only important to diagnose those comorbid conditions early, but also vital to treat those conditions appropriately, which may have a huge impact on the primary disease itself. The common conditions are discussed in this review, but there are multiple other comorbidities beyond the scope of this article. The physician should try treating "patients as a whole" instead of treating the specific disease, and this approach may require multidisciplinary care.

Heart failure (HF) and atrial fibrillation (AF) are highly prevalent debilitating conditions that often coexist and are frequently encountered in clinical practice. The presence of chronic AF is a marker of worse prognosis in patients with HF, and the onset of new AF in those with chronic HF is associated with increased morbidity and mortality. Advances in the development of novel drugs, nonpharmacologic modalities, and therapeutic strategies, as well the increased understanding of the pathobiology of HF and AF, are key to mitigating the tremendous public health burden that is associated with these conditions.

The prevalence of chemotherapy-related cardiac disease is increasing because of patient survivorship and the development of novel chemotherapies that may be cardiotoxic. Management requires a multidisciplinary approach from cardiologists and oncologists. Pretreatment identification of predisposing risk factors and assessment of cardiac function before and at intervals during and after therapy with cardiotoxic agents are necessary. In clinical practice, surveillance is largely performed using transthoracic echocardiography or multi-gated radionuclide angiography. Imaging strategies that detect cardiac injury before overt left ventricular systolic dysfunction provide an opportunity for early intervention and improved cardiac outcomes.

Preface

Heart Failure: A Common and Complex Clinical Syndrome

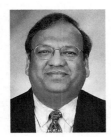

Prakash C. Deedwania, MD, FACC, FACP, FASH, FAHA
Guest Editor

This issue of *Medical Clinics of North America* focuses on various issues dealing with heart failure (HF). It is quite evident to most clinicians that HF is a major growing public health problem. Most clinicians frequently encounter patients with HF in everyday clinical practice. HF is a leading cause for hospitalization (≥ 1 million admissions yearly) in the Medicare population. Appropriate treatment designed to prevent and treat heart failure can significantly reduce the associated high morbidity and mortality. It is with this focus that I have put together this compendium of articles dealing with the most important issues regarding the pathophysiology, diagnosis, and treatment of patients with HF and frequently associated comorbidities.

In the first article we describe the current epidemiology and focus on the renewed understanding of the pathophysiologic process involved in various stages of the development of HF. A clear understanding of the pathophysiology should help the clinician target appropriate therapy. The second article by Dr Chatterjee describes the differences and similarities between the signs, symptoms, and prognostic factors in systolic versus diastolic HF. This is particularly important due to the fact that, depending on the clinical setting, as many as one half of the patients with HF nowadays have diastolic HF (also known as HF with preserved ejection fraction). The advent of biomarkers, especially BNP, has revolutionized the diagnostic accuracy for HF and this along with the value of other biomarkers in HF is discussed in detail in the article by Maisel and coauthors.

During the past 2 decades considerable progress has been made regarding the use of evidence-based therapy with RAAS blocking agents (ACE inhibitors, ARBs, and aldosterone antagonists) and β-blocking drugs in HF. Treatment with these drugs is now recommended by all national and international guidelines as standard therapy in HF. Such evidence-based therapy not only improves symptoms but also reduces the morbidity and mortality in patients with HF, which is described in detail in article 4.

Although diuretic therapy is extremely useful in relieving congestion, it is considered by many as the standard treatment in all patients with HF. It is important to recognize

Med Clin N Am 96 (2012) xi–xii
http://dx.doi.org/10.1016/j.mcna.2012.08.001
0025-7125/12/$ – see front matter Published by Elsevier Inc.

medical.theclinics.com

that diuretics need to be used only in the setting of a fluid-overloaded state and that excessive and unnecessary use of diuretics can lead to further activation of neurohormonal axes and in some cases the development of cardiorenal syndrome. We describe the underlying mechanism and appropriate use of diuretic therapy along with discussion of some new diuretics in article 5.

Many patients with HF have symptoms and signs related to low cardiac output and often require inotropic therapy to maintain adequate perfusion. However, despite the necessity to use inotropes in HF, a number of studies have demonstrated that there is increased mortality associated with the use of inotropic therapy and hence it is crucial to understand appropriate uses and limitations of such treatment. These issues are discussed in detail in article 6 by Hauptman and coauthors. As mentioned earlier, inappropriate and excessive use of diuretics can lead to cardiorenal syndrome. Additionally, this issue is compounded by underlying CKD that is present in as many as one third of patients with HF. The underlying pathophysiology and management of patients with cardiorenal syndrome is discussed in detail by Butler and associates in article 7.

The next article by Tang and coauthors deals with the frequent issues of comorbidities such as diabetes, anemia, etc, that are frequently encountered in patients with HF and have significant impact on the prognosis as well as management of patients with HF. Atrial fibrillation and heart failure often coexist and each has a significant impact on the management issues and prognosis of the other. During the past decade there have been several pivotal studies that have evaluated the impact of various therapeutic strategies in patients with HF and atrial fibrillation. These are discussed in detail in the article by Lardizabal. Finally, HF in cancer patients often related to chemotherapy use is discussed in detail by Moslehi and coworkers.

Although it is difficult to cover everything about HF and related conditions in a limited monograph such as this one, I have attempted to include the topics that are most relevant for the clinician in everyday practice in the hope that expanding their knowledge in these areas will improve patient care and curb the growing burden of HF in clinical practice. The articles included in this monograph have been written by authors who have considerable expertise in the given areas and have made a lot of effort in synthesizing complex and extensive literature to prepare their reviews. I would like to acknowledge their sincere efforts and time commitment in preparing their excellent contributions to this monograph. I would also like to thank Pamela Hetherington for her efforts in coordinating this issue in a timely manner. Finally, I would like to thank all my residents and fellows, as well as patients, who are a constant source of inspiration.

Prakash C. Deedwania, MD, FACC, FACP, FASH, FAHA
Professor, School of Medicine
University of California-San Francisco
San Francisco, CA, USA

Cardiology Division
Veterans Affairs Central California System
VACCHS Medical Center
2515 East Clinton Avenue
Fresno, CA 93703, USA

E-mail address:
deed@fresno.ucsf.edu

The Epidemiology and Pathophysiology of Heart Failure

Shradha Rathi, MD[a], Prakash C. Deedwania, MD[b],*

KEYWORDS

- Heart failure • Epidemiology • Pathophysiology • Hospitalization

KEY POINTS

- In the medicare population, heart failure is the leading cause for hospitalization, accounting for >1 million admissions per year.
- Triggered by myocardial insult, maladaptive neurohumoral processes including the sympathetic (adrenergic) nervous system and the renin-angiotensin-aldosterone system, result in an ever-spiraling deterioration of cardiovascular function and cardiac remodeling.

INTRODUCTION

Heart failure (HF) remains a major growing public health problem in the United States. Despite extensive understanding of the mechanism at the molecular level and innovations in therapy, HF carries high morbidity and mortality rates, with frequent hospital admissions. In the Medicare population, HF is the leading cause for hospitalization, accounting for more than 1 million admissions per year. The authors review the epidemiology and pathophysiology of HF.

EPIDEMIOLOGY

The prevalence of HF is estimated to be 5.7 million on the basis of the latest data from the National Health and Nutrition Examination Study (NHANES) 2005 to 2008 as mentioned in "Heart Disease and Stroke Statistics–2012 Update: A Report from the American Heart Association."[1] Projections of crude prevalence show that in 2010, approximately 6.6 million (2.8%) US adults older than 18 years had HF.[2] It is estimated that by 2030, an additional 3 million people will have HF, representing a 25.0% increase in prevalence from 2010.[2] Data from the National Heart, Lung, and Blood Institute–sponsored Framingham Heart Study (FHS)[3] indicate that HF incidence approaches 10 cases/1000 population after age 65 years. Seventy-five percent of

[a] Cardiology Department, UCSF Fresno Cardiology, 2823 North Fresno Street, 5th Floor, Fresno, CA 93721, USA; [b] Cardiology Division, Veterans Affairs Central California Health Care System, University of California at San Francisco, 2615 East Clinton Avenue, E224, Fresno, CA 93703, USA
* Corresponding author.
E-mail address: deed@fresno.ucsf.edu

Med Clin N Am 96 (2012) 881–890
http://dx.doi.org/10.1016/j.mcna.2012.07.011
0025-7125/12/$ – see front matter Published by Elsevier Inc.

medical.theclinics.com

patients with HF have antecedent hypertension. At age 40 years, the lifetime risk of developing HF for men and women is 1:5. At age 80 years, the remaining lifetime risk for the development of new HF is 20% for men and women, even in the face of a much shorter life expectancy. At age 40 years, the lifetime risk of HF occurring without antecedent myocardial infarction (MI) is 1:9 for men and 1:6 for women. The lifetime risk for people with blood pressure (BP) greater than 160/90 mm Hg is twice that for people with BP less than 140/90 mm Hg. The annual rates of new HF events/1000 population for white men are 15.2 cases for those aged 65 to 74 years, 31.7 cases for those aged 75 to 84 years, and 65.2 cases for those older than 85 years. For white women in the same age groups, the rates are 8.2, 19.8, and 45.6 cases/1000 population, respectively. For black men in the same age groups, the rates are 16.9, 25.5, and 50.6 cases/1000 population, and for black women in the same age groups, the estimated rates are 14.2, 25.5, and 44.0 cases/1000 population, respectively (Community Health Study [CHS], National Heart, Lung and Blood Institute [NHLBI]). In (multi ethic study of atherosclerosis [MESA]), African Americans had the highest risk of developing HF, followed by Hispanic, white, and Chinese Americans (4.6, 3.5, 2.4, and 1.0 case/1000 person-years, respectively). This higher risk reflected differences in the prevalence of hypertension and diabetes mellitus and in socioeconomic status. African Americans had the highest proportion of incident HF not preceded by clinical MI (75%).[4] Survival after HF diagnosis has improved, as shown by data from the FHS[5] and the Olmsted County Study.[6] However, overall mortality remains high: approximately 50% of people diagnosed with HF will die within 5 years.[6,7] In the National Heart, Lung, and Blood Institute–sponsored FHS, hypertension was found to be the most common population-attributable risk factor for HF, followed closely by antecedent MI.[8] Among 20 900 male physicians in the Physicians Health Study, the lifetime risk of HF was higher in men with hypertension; healthy lifestyle factors (eg, normal weight, not smoking, regular exercise, moderate alcohol intake, consumption of breakfast cereals, and consumption of fruits and vegetables) were related to lower risk of HF.[9]

HF is one of the leading causes of hospitalization in the United States. Among 1077 patients with HF in Olmsted County, MN, USA, hospitalizations were common after HF diagnosis (mean age 76.8 years, 54.0% female) during a mean follow-up of 4.7 years. After HF diagnosis, 83.1% patients were hospitalized at least once, and 43% were hospitalized at least 4 times. The reason for hospitalization was HF in 16.5% and other cardiovascular causes in 21.6%, whereas more than half (61.9%) of reasons for hospitalization were noncardiovascular. Male sex, diabetes mellitus, chronic obstructive pulmonary disease, anemia, and creatinine clearance less than 30 mL/min were independent predictors of hospitalization (P<.05 for each).[10] These data clearly indicate that HF is a major contributor to health care expenditure. It is likely that the prevalence of HF will increase further because of the aging of the US population and the improved survival of those with acute MI, hypertension, and other cardiovascular conditions. It is only with the implementation of preventative strategies that the incidence of HF will decrease, but until then it is safe to assume that HF will continue to remain a major contributor to increased morbidity and mortality in cardiac patients.

PATHOPHYSIOLOGY OF HF

HF is a progressive, complex clinical syndrome that can result from any structural or functional cardiac injury that impairs the ability of the ventricle to fill with or eject blood. It represents a profound derangement of otherwise fine-tuned physiologic mechanisms to maintain cardiac output, BP, and fluid balance. In the absence of injury, the normal adult heart is a stable mechanical tissue pump adjusting performance to changes in loading conditions and inotropic state. Myocardial injury alters the loading and biochemical environment of both impaired and uninjured cardiac cells. Endocrine, paracrine (on neighboring cells), autocrine (on the same cell), or intracrine (internally on the same cell without extracellular secretion) mechanisms all can contribute to a subsequent net biologic response.[11] As in other tissues, these signals potentially reinitiate a fetal growth repertoire of transcription and translation.[12,13] Over time, characteristic patterns of cardiac morphology emerge, leading to the progression of ventricular systolic and/or diastolic impairment. The pathophysiology of systolic and diastolic HF is also discussed elsewhere in this issue by Chatterjee and colleagues. Shifts in the physical characteristics of the heart require an orchestrated sequence of cell proliferation, apoptosis, hypertrophy, and atrophy—a process referred to as ventricular remodeling.[12] Cardiac remodeling process has been attributed to a variety of cellular mechanisms that are activated with cardiac dysfunction. Next, the authors discuss the role of neuroendocrine mechanisms in detail.

NEUROHORMONAL RESPONSE IN HF

With myocardial injury, several compensatory mechanisms are activated, including the adrenergic nervous system and renin-angiotensin-aldosterone system (RAAS), responsible for maintaining cardiac output through increased retention of salt and water, peripheral arterial vasoconstriction, and increased contractility. In addition, inflammatory mediators, which are responsible for cardiac repair and remodeling, are activated. Although these neuroendocrine mechanisms are compensatory during the acute adaptive phase, their continued activation is deleterious and propagates further cardiac dysfunction, a chronic maladaptive phase.

SYMPATHETIC NERVOUS SYSTEM

One of the most important adaptive responses to cardiac dysfunction is activation of the sympathetic (adrenergic) nervous system, which occurs early in the course of HF. Although these disturbances in autonomic control were initially attributed to loss of the inhibitory input from arterial or cardiopulmonary baroreceptor reflexes, there is increasing evidence that excitatory reflexes also participate in the autonomic imbalance that occurs in HF.[14] Under normal conditions, inhibitory inputs from the high-pressure carotid sinus and aortic arch baroreceptors and the low-pressure cardiopulmonary mechanoreceptors are the principal inhibitors of sympathetic outflow, whereas discharges from the nonbaroreflex peripheral chemoreceptors and muscle metaboreceptors are the major excitatory inputs to sympathetic outflow. The vagal limb of the baroreceptor heart rate reflex is also responsive to arterial baroreceptor afferent inhibitory input. Healthy individuals display low sympathetic discharge at rest and have high heart rate variability. However, in patients with HF, inhibitory input from baroreceptors and mechanoreceptors decreases and excitatory input increases, with the net result that there is a generalized increase in sympathetic nerve traffic and blunted parasympathetic nerve traffic, with the resultant loss of heart rate variability and increased peripheral vascular resistance.[14] The major marker of sympathetic nervous system activity is increased norepinephrine (NE) levels; epinephrine levels are not significantly elevated in HF. As a result of the increase in sympathetic tone, there is an increase in circulating levels of NE, a potent adrenergic neurotransmitter. Coronary sinus NE levels are many times higher than arterial levels, and increased levels are also seen in renal veins.[15] The elevated levels of circulating NE result from a combination of increased release of NE from adrenergic nerve endings and its consequent "spillover" into the plasma, with reduced uptake of NE by adrenergic nerve endings. In patients with advanced HF, the circulating levels of NE in resting patients are 2 to 3 times those found in normal subjects. Indeed, plasma levels of NE predict mortality in patients with HF.

Stimulation of the sympathetic nervous system with release of NE has widespread physiologic effects. In normal individuals or patients in the early stages of HF, NE increases heart rate and contractility and may support cardiac function. However, in later stages of cardiac decompensation, cardiac response to NE is blunted, partly because of the decreased β-receptor density seen in patients with chronic severe HF.[16] There is a shift from the normal β-adrenergic receptor density in a β_1-to-β_2 ratio of 70% to 80%/20% to 30% to a more even distribution of 60%/40%. α-Receptors increase in the failing heart so that the end result is a more balanced distribution of α-, β_1-, and β_2-receptors. Decreased β-receptor density could conceivably contribute to reduced cardiac function in HF.

Genetic variations in β-receptor subtypes also are related to the risk of developing HF. African Americans who are homozygous for a variant of the α_2-receptor are 5 times more likely to develop HF.[17]

Peripheral arteriolar tone is increased, producing an elevation of BP and cardiac afterload via α-receptor activation. In the kidney, however, activation of the sympathetic nervous system causes significant sodium retention via disproportionate vasoconstriction of the efferent arterioles.[18] The resulting increased pressure in the glomerulus helps to maintain glomerular filtration rate but favors the reabsorption of sodium and water in the proximal tubule.[19] In addition, sympathetic stimulation increases production of rennin, angiotensin II, and aldosterone, promoting even further sodium reabsorption.[20] Beyond the detrimental hemodynamic effects of the sympathetic nervous system, there is evidence that NE itself produces direct detrimental effects at the cardiac level. High circulating levels of NE strongly correlate with left ventricular dysfunction and mortality.[21,22] Direct exposure to myocytes in tissue culture to levels of NE that are seen in HF results in cell death with increased intracellular calcium levels.[23] Communal and associates[24] showed that NE induced cardiac apoptosis in rat adult myocytes, acting through protein kinase, and was independent of β-adrenergic receptors. Cardiac fibrosis is also promoted by NE acting via transforming growth factor β1.[25]

RAAS

The RAAS plays a key role in regulating electrolyte levels and fluid balance in normal physiology. Increased renin production by the kidney in patients with HF was shown in the 1940s.[26] RAAS is activated relatively later in HF. The presumptive mechanisms for renin-angiotensin system (RAS) activation in HF include renal hypoperfusion, decreased filtered sodium reaching the macula densa in the distal tubule causing decreased stretch of the juxtaglomerular apparatus or its stimulation by the sympathetic nervous system increases renin release.[27] Renin cleaves 4 amino acids from circulating angiotensinogen, which is synthesized in the liver to form the biologically inactive decapeptide angiotensin I. Angiotensin-converting enzyme (ACE) cleaves 2 amino acids from angiotensin I to form the biologically active octapeptide (1–8) angiotensin II, which is a key substrate to couple with angiotensin 1 receptors, and subsequently causes vasoconstriction and vascular and cardiac remodeling and leads to salt and water retention via the release of aldosterone. In the kidney, angiotensin II causes vasoconstriction in the large-bore muscular renal arteries but predominantly in the efferent (postglomerular) arterioles.[28] The vasoconstriction produces higher pressure in the glomerulus and filtration of fluid and electrolytes, which pass into the proximal tubule. The lower hydrostatic pressure and increased oncotic pressure in the postglomerular vessels surrounding the proximal tubule promote reabsorption of sodium and water. Urea is passively reabsorbed along with water, whereas creatinine is not reabsorbed, leading to the high blood urea nitrogen/creatinine ratios seen in some patients with HF. Increased circulating levels of angiotensin II promote the release of aldosterone from the zona glomerulosa of the adrenal gland, which also results in sodium reabsorption in the distal nephron and potassium excretion.[29] Finally, angiotensin II may increase the release of arginine vasopressin via a mechanism that does not rely on changes in osmolality.[30] This nonosmotic release of vasopressin is partly responsible for hyponatremia seen with severe HF. A tissue-based RAS has also been discovered, which contributes both positively and negatively to the HF syndrome.[31] Locally produced angiotensin II increases cardiac contractility, which may help to compensate initially for myocardial injury. This effect may be mediated by increased NE release from the presynaptic nerve endings.[32] Local angiotensin II initiates the production of growth factors and has been shown to cause myocyte hypertrophy and ultimately left ventricular hypertrophy.[33] Collagen production is also increased, which, along with sodium retention and venoconstriction caused by angiotensin II, brings about increased filling pressures that are responsible for many features of chronic HF. High aldosterone levels are also associated with myocardial fibrosis.[34] Angiotensin II is produced within the vascular bed and by cytokine-stimulated monocytes.

Although the use of angiotensin-converting enzyme inhibitors (ACEIs) reduces the production of angiotensin II, there are alternative pathways for its formation so that angiotensin II levels are not suppressed completely with ACEIs. This has been termed "ACEI escape" through the enzymatic conversion of angiotensinogen to angiotensin I by kallikrein and cathepsin G and may permit continued production of angiotensin II despite ACE inhibition. The tissue production of angiotensin II may also occur through ACE-independent pathways, through the activation of chymase; this pathway may be of major importance in the myocardium, particularly when the levels of renin and angiotensin I are increased by the use of ACEIs. Although angiotensin receptor blockers can theoretically overcome this problem via direct blockade of the angiotensin I receptor activity regardless of the mechanism of their activation, the use of angiotensin receptor blockers either alone or in combination with ACEIs has not consistently shown improved outcomes in HF.[35,36] Based on these data, it can be concluded that alterations in the sympathoadrenal axis is a major player in the pathophysiologic process involved in HF.

NATRIURETIC PEPTIDES

Discovered slightly more than 50 years ago as secretory granules in the atria, the natriuretic peptides have been the object of intense scientific study.[37] The role of natriuretic peptide as a marker for HF is being discussed elsewhere in this issue by Maisel and colleagues. Here, the authors discuss the role of natriuretic peptides in the pathophysiology of HF. The natriuretic peptides (atrial natriuretic peptide and B-type natriuretic peptide [BNP]) bind to a specific transmembrane receptor called NPR-A (natriuretic peptide receptor-A) that results in the production of guanosine monophosphate.[38] The synthesis and release of BNP correlate with increased ventricular wall stress. Infusion of BNP produces prompt reduction of right atrial, pulmonary artery, and pulmonary artery wedge pressures.[39] In addition, systemic vascular resistance declines and cardiac output improves with increased natriuretic peptide levels.[40,41] In acute infusion studies, BNP is associated with reduced circulating aldosterone and decreases NE levels in the coronary sinus of individuals with systolic dysfunction.[42,43]

The data on renal effects are less consistent in HF. In animal models and in individuals without cardiac dysfunction, BNP produces natriuresis and an increase in glomerular filtration rate.[44,45] These effects have been shown in some studies in patients with HF but not in other studies.[45,46] A meta-analysis of early BNP infusion trials showed an increased risk of worsening renal function at 30 days.[47] Despite high circulating levels of natriuretic peptides that have been consistently shown in HF and their antagonistic effects on deleterious neurohormonal activation, the syndrome persists. The reasons are unclear, but several potential explanations have been suggested. The profound activation of the RAS and sympathetic nervous system may overcome the ability of natriuretic peptides to increase sodium excretion or reduce afterload. An alternative explanation for which there are new data from research with the use of mass spectroscopy is that circulating natriuretic peptides are not biologically active.[48]

Ventricular Remodeling

Myocardial injury alters the loading and biochemical environment of both impaired and uninjured cardiac cells. Endocrine, paracrine, autocrine, or intracrine mechanisms all can contribute to a subsequent net biologic response.[11] As in other tissues, these signals potentially reinitiate a fetal growth series of transcription and translation.[12,13] Over time, characteristic patterns of cardiac morphology emerge associated with the progression of ventricular systolic or diastolic impairment. Shifts in the physical characteristics of the heart require an orchestrated sequence of cell proliferation, apoptosis, hypertrophy, and atrophy—a process referred to as ventricular remodeling.[13] Although remodeling may represent a reparative response to abnormal myocardial conditions, it generally contributes to ventricular dysfunction when fully manifest and is persistent in the long term.

In 1975, Grossman and coworkers[49] proposed the hypothesis that increased wall stress initiates concentric or eccentric hypertrophy until regional wall stress returns to normal. Other components triggering hypertrophy could include stretch of the sarcomere-spanning protein titin and modulation of other growth factors.[50] The extracellular environment provides scaffolding for and participates in differentiation of cardiac muscle and nonmuscle cells.[51] Extracellular matrix modifications[52] also are important components of ventricular remodeling. After ischemic or nonischemic insults, increased deposition of fibrous proteins including collagen and fibronectin contributes to the altered mechanical properties of the remodeled left ventricle.[53,54] These alterations are promulgated by activation of the RAAS. Its stimulation, and the spillover of aldosterone, is responsible for extracellular matrix proliferation and contributes to the increased deposition of fibrous tissue within the ventricular myocardium. The presence of myocardial fibrosis and endothelial dysfunction may affect the coronary microcirculation; in particular, the decrease in myocardial capillary density can contribute to the progression of left ventricular remodeling toward HF. For this and other reasons, therapeutic interventions in patients with post-MI left ventricular dysfunction are aimed at preventing the activation of the RAAS, with possible beneficial effects on left ventricular structure, size, and function. ACEIs were the first drugs used to block the RAAS. Inhibition of ACE results in a decrease in the concentration of angiotensin II at the angiotensin receptor sites. During the past 30 years, several clinical trials have demonstrated the beneficial effects of ACEIs in patients with acute MI, with favorable prognostic implications. The Survival And Ventricular Enlargement (SAVE) trial was a landmark study by Pfeiffer and colleagues.[55] They enrolled patients with left ventricular dysfunction (ejection fraction no greater than 40%) after acute MI, who were treated with captopril, starting between 3 and 16 days after admission to hospital. An attenuation of ventricular enlargement became apparent after 12 months and was associated with a significant reduction in morbidity and mortality.

Compared with a normal ventricle, a failing left ventricle may be characterized by systolic or diastolic dysfunction, or both, graphically represented by alterations in pressure-volume characteristics of the left ventricular chamber. Typically, a primary decrease in systolic function is associated with a small initial increase in heart size. Subsequently, secondary ventricular remodeling can lead to marked changes in heart size and function, causing the normal ellipsoid form to become globular. Right ventricular dysfunction can contribute to the HF syndrome. The most common cause of right HF is left HF.[56] If right HF seems out of proportion to left HF, primary myocardial disorders, including systemic diseases such as sarcoidosis or amyloidosis, should be considered.[57] It is often difficult to ascertain in individual patients when primary injury and secondary adverse myocardial remodeling[58] have progressed to a state refractory to medical intervention. Systemic factors may be as important as measurable cardiac parameters.[59] With chronic unloading in patients such as occurs after left ventricular assist device implantation, reverse remodeling can return diastolic pressure-volume relationships to normal.[60] Nevertheless, improvement of systolic function adequate to permit device explantation is uncommon.[61] With left ventricular assist device placement in patients with nonischemic HF, the potential for recovery of left ventricular systolic function seems to be progressively reduced as diastolic dimension[62] and histologic myocyte hypertrophy and fibrosis increase.[63]

SUMMARY

HF remains a challenging, relentless health condition associated with millions of rehospitalizations annually. Triggered by myocardial insult, maladaptive neurohumoral processes, including the sympathetic (adrenergic) nervous system and RAAS, result in an ever-spiraling deterioration of cardiovascular function and cardiac remodeling. A clear understanding of the pathways involved in the pathophysiology of HF will be helpful in the application of appropriate therapy for patients in the clinic with HF.

REFERENCES

1. Roger VL, Go AS, Lloyd-Jones D, et al. Heart disease and stroke statistics–2012 update: a report from the American Heart Association. Circulation 2012;125: e2–220.
2. Heidenreich PA, Trogdon JG, Khavjou OA, et al. Forecasting the future of cardiovascular disease in the United States: a policy statement from the American Heart Association. Circulation 2011;123:933–44.
3. Lloyd-Jones D, Larson MG, Leip EP, et al. Lifetime risk for developing congestive heart failure: the Framingham Heart Study. Circulation 2002;106:3068–72.
4. Bahrami H, Kronmal R, Bluemke DA, et al. Differences in the incidence of congestive heart failure by ethnicity: the multi-ethnic study of atherosclerosis. Arch Intern Med 2008;168:2138–45.
5. Matsushita K, Blecker S, Pazin-Filho A, et al. The association of hemoglobin A1c with incident heart failure among people without diabetes: the Atherosclerosis Risk in Communities Study. Diabetes 2010;59:2020–6.
6. Roger VL, Weston SA, Redfield MM, et al. Trends in heart failure incidence and survival in a community-based population. JAMA 2004;292:344–50.

7. Levy D, Kenchaiah S, Larson MG, et al. Long-term trends in the incidence of and survival with heart failure. N Engl J Med 2002;347:1397–402.

8. Velagaleti RS, Gona P, Larson MG, et al. Multimarker approach for the prediction of heart failure incidence in the community. Circulation 2010;122:1700–6.

9. Djoussé L, Driver JA, Gaziano JM. Relation between modifiable lifestyle factors and lifetime risk of heart failure. JAMA 2009;302:394–400.

10. Dunlay SM, Redfield MM, Weston SA, et al. Hospitalizations after heart failure diagnosis a community perspective. J Am Coll Cardiol 2009;54:1695–702.

11. Lionetti V, Bianchi G, Recchia FA, et al. Control of autocrine and paracrine myocardial signals: an emerging therapeutic strategy in heart failure. Heart Fail Rev 2010;15:531–42.

12. Mann DL, Bristow MR. Mechanisms and models in heart failure: the biomechanical model and beyond. Circulation 2005;111:2837–49.

13. Yang R, Amir J, Liu H, et al. Mechanical strain activates a program of genes functionally involved in paracrine signaling of angiogenesis. Physiol Genomics 2008; 36:1–14.

14. Floras JS. Sympathetic activation in human heart failure: diverse mechanisms, therapeutic opportunities. Acta Physiol Scand 2003;177:391–8.

15. Swedberg K, Viquerat C, Rouleau JL, et al. Comparison of myocardial catecholamine balance in chronic congestive heart failure and in angina pectoris without failure. Am J Cardiol 1984;54:783–6.

16. Bristow MR, Ginsburg R, Minobe W, et al. Decreased catecholamine sensitivity and beta-adrenergic-receptor density in failing human hearts. N Engl J Med 1982;307:205–11.

17. Bristow MR, Ginsburg R, Umans V, et al. Beta 1- and beta 2-adrenergic-receptor subpopulations in nonfailing and failing human ventricular myocardium: coupling of both receptor subtypes to muscle contraction and selective beta 1-receptor down-regulation in heart failure. Circ Res 1986;59:297–309.

18. Ichikawa I, Pfeffer JM, Pfeffer MA, et al. Role of angiotensin II in the altered renal function of congestive heart failure. Circ Res 1984;55:669–75.

19. Bell-Reuss E, Trevino DL, Gottschalk CW. Effect of renal sympathetic nerve stimulation on proximal water and sodium reabsorption. J Clin Invest 1976;57:1104–7.

20. McLeod AA, Brown JE, Kuhn C, et al. Differentiation of hemodynamic, humoral and metabolic responses to beta 1- and beta 2-adrenergic stimulation in man using atenolol and propranolol. Circulation 1983;67:1076–84.

21. Francis GS, Goldsmith SR, Cohn JN. Relationship of exercise capacity to resting left ventricular performance and basal plasma norepinephrine levels in patients with congestive heart failure. Am Heart J 1982;104:725–31.

22. Cohn JN, Levine TB, Olivari MT, et al. Plasma norepinephrine as a guide to prognosis in patients with chronic congestive heart failure. N Engl J Med 1984;311: 819–23.

23. Mann DL, Kent RL, Parsons B, et al. Adrenergic effects on the biology of the adult mammalian cardiocyte. Circulation 1992;85:790–804.

24. Communal C, Singh K, Pimentel DR, et al. Norepinephrine stimulates apoptosis in adult rat ventricular myocytes by activation of the beta-adrenergic pathway. Circulation 1998;98:1329–34.

25. Lijnen PJ, Petrov VV, Fagard RH. Induction of cardiac fibrosis by transforming growth factor-beta(1). Mol Genet Metab 2000;71:418–35.

26. Merrill AJ, Morrison JL, Branno ES. Concentration of renin in renal venous blood in patients with chronic heart failure. Am J Med 1946;1:468.

27. Davis JO. The control of renin release. Am J Med 1973;55:333–50.

28. Hall JE, Coleman TG, Guyton AC, et al. Intrarenal role of angiotensin II and [des-Asp1]angiotensin II. Am J Physiol 1979;236:F252–9.
29. Pratt JH. Role of angiotensin II in potassium-mediated stimulation of aldosterone secretion in the dog. J Clin Invest 1982;70:667–72.
30. Ishikawa S, Saito T, Yoshida S. The effect of osmotic pressure and angiotensin II on arginine vasopressin release from guinea pig hypothalamo-neurohypophyseal complex in organ culture. Endocrinology 1980;106:1571–8.
31. Hirsch AT, Talsness CE, Schunkert H, et al. Tissue-specific activation of cardiac angiotensin converting enzyme in experimental heart failure. Circ Res 1991;69:475–82.
32. Burgdorf C, Richardt D, Kurz T, et al. Presynaptic regulation of norepinephrine release in a model of nonfailing hypertrophied myocardium. J Cardiovasc Pharmacol 2003;41:813–6.
33. Sadoshima J, Izumo S. Molecular characterization of angiotensin II–induced hypertrophy of cardiac myocytes and hyperplasia of cardiac fibroblasts. Critical role of the AT1 receptor subtype. Circ Res 1993;73:413–23.
34. Weber KT, Brilla CG. Pathological hypertrophy and cardiac interstitium. Fibrosis and renin-angiotensin-aldosterone system. Circulation 1991;83:1849–65.
35. Cohn JN, Tognoni G, Valsartan Heart Failure Trial Investigators. A randomized trial of the angiotensin-receptor blocker valsartan in chronic heart failure. N Engl J Med 2001;345:1667–75.
36. McMurray JJ, Ostergren J, Swedberg K, et al. Effects of candesartan in patients with chronic heart failure and reduced left-ventricular systolic function taking angiotensin-converting-enzyme inhibitors: the CHARM-added trial. Lancet 2003;362:767–71.
37. Kisch B. Electron microscopic investigations of the heart of cattle. 1. The atrium of the heart of cows. Exp Med Surg 1959;17:247–61.
38. Levin ER, Gardner DG, Samson WK. Natriuretic peptides. N Engl J Med 1998;339:321–8.
39. Iwanaga Y, Nishi I, Furuichi S, et al. B-type natriuretic peptide strongly reflects diastolic wall stress in patients with chronic heart failure: comparison between systolic and diastolic heart failure. J Am Coll Cardiol 2006;47:742–8.
40. Yoshimura M, Yasue H, Morita E, et al. Hemodynamic, renal, and hormonal responses to brain natriuretic peptide infusion in patients with congestive heart failure. Circulation 1991;84:1581–8.
41. Marcus LS, Hart D, Packer M, et al. Hemodynamic and renal excretory effects of human brain natriuretic peptide infusion in patients with congestive heart failure. A double-blind, placebo-controlled, randomized crossover trial. Circulation 1996;94:3184–9.
42. Abraham WT, Lowes BD, Ferguson DA, et al. Systemic hemodynamic, neurohormonal, and renal effects of a steady-state infusion of human brain natriuretic peptide in patients with hemodynamically decompensated heart failure. J Card Fail 1998;4:37–44.
43. Brunner-La Rocca HP, Kaye DM, Woods RL, et al. Effects of intravenous brain natriuretic peptide on regional sympathetic activity in patients with chronic heart failure as compared with healthy control subjects. J Am Coll Cardiol 2001;37:1221–7.
44. Marin-Grez M, Fleming JT, Steinhausen M. Atrial natriuretic peptide causes preglomerular vasodilatation and post-glomerular vasoconstriction in rat kidney. Nature 1986;324:473–6.
45. La Villa G, Fronzaroli C, Lazzeri C, et al. Cardiovascular and renal effects of low dose brain natriuretic peptide infusion in man. J Clin Endocrinol Metab 1994;78:1166–71.

46. Jensen KT, Eiskjaer H, Carstens J, et al. Renal effects of brain natriuretic peptide in patients with congestive heart failure. Clin Sci (Lond) 1999;96:5–15.

47. Sackner-Bernstein J, Skopicki HA, Aaronson KD. Risk of worsening renal function with nesiritide in patients with acutely decompensated heart failure. Circulation 2005;111:1487–91.

48. Hawkridge AM, Heublein DM, Bergen HR, et al. Quantitative mass spectral evidence for the absence of circulating brain natriuretic peptide (BNP-32) in severe human heart failure. Proc Natl Acad Sci U S A 2005;102:17442–7.

49. Grossman W, Jones D, McLaurin LP. Wall stress and patterns of hypertrophy in the human left ventricle. J Clin Invest 1975;56:56–64.

50. Linke WA. Sense and stretchability: the role of titin and titin-associated proteins in myocardial stress-sensing and mechanical dysfunction. Cardiovasc Res 2008; 77:637–48.

51. Deschamps AM, Spinale FG. Disruptions and detours in the myocardial matrix highway and heart failure. Curr Heart Fail Rep 2005;2:10–7.

52. Weber KT. Extracellular matrix remodeling in heart failure: a role for de novo angiotensin II generation. Circulation 1997;96:4065–82.

53. Borer JS, Truter S, Herrold EM, et al. Myocardial fibrosis in chronic aortic regurgitation: molecular and cellular responses to volume overload. Circulation 2002;105:1837–42.

54. Jugdutt BI. Ventricular remodeling after infarction and the extracellular collagen matrix: when is enough enough? Circulation 2003;108:1395–403.

55. Pfeffer MA, Braunwald E, Moye LA, et al. Effect of captopril on mortality and morbidity in patients with left ventricular dysfunction after myocardial infarction. results of the Survival And Ventricular Enlargement Trial. The SAVE Investigators. N Engl J Med 1992;327(10):669–77.

56. Thibault GE. Clinical problem-solving. Studying the classics. N Engl J Med 1995; 333:648–52.

57. Seward JB, Casaclang-Verzosa G. Infiltrative cardiovascular diseases: cardiomyopathies that look alike. J Am Coll Cardiol 2010;55:1769–79.

58. Gorlin R. Treatment of congestive heart failure: where are we going? Circulation 1987;75:IV108–11.

59. Levy WC, Mozaffarian D, Linker DT, et al. The Seattle Heart Failure Model: prediction of survival in heart failure. Circulation 2006;113:1424–33.

60. Levin HR, Oz MC, Chen JM, et al. Reversal of chronic ventricular dilation in patients with end-stage cardiomyopathy by prolonged mechanical unloading. Circulation 1995;91:2717–20.

61. Miller LW, Pagani FD, Russell SD, et al. Use of a continuous-flow device in patients awaiting heart transplantation. N Engl J Med 2007;357:885–96.

62. Simon MA, Primack BA, Teuteberg J, et al. Left ventricular remodeling and myocardial recovery on mechanical circulatory support. J Card Fail 2010;16: 99–105.

63. Saito S, Matsumiya G, Sakaguchi T, et al. Cardiac fibrosis and cellular hypertrophy decrease the degree of reverse remodeling and improvement in cardiac function during left ventricular assist. J Heart Lung Transplant 2010;29:672–9.

Pathophysiology of Systolic and Diastolic Heart Failure

Kanu Chatterjee, MB, FRCP(Lond), FRCP (Edin), FCCP, MACP

KEYWORDS

- Chronic heart failure • Systolic heart failure • Diastolic heart failure

KEY POINTS

- Systolic and diastolic heart failure are the 2 most common clinical subsets of chronic heart failure.
- Left ventricular "Starling" function is depressed in patients with systolic heart failure.
- In systolic heart failure, left ventricular mass is increased, which can be measured by transthoracic echocardiography. Cardiac magnetic resonance imaging is a more precise technique to measure left ventricular mass.
- Neurohormonal activation is a major pathophysiologic mechanism for ventricular remodeling and progression of heart failure in systolic heart failure.

HISTORICAL PERSPECTIVES

The differences between systolic and diastolic heart failure have been recognized for several decades. In 1937, Dr Fishberg described that diastolic heart failure results from inadequate ventricular filling, and he termed this type of heart failure as hypodiastolic failure. He also recognized that systolic heart failure results from inadequate emptying of the heart and he called it hyposystolic failure.[1]

Definitions

The most commonly used definition of systolic heart failure is that "it is a pathophysiologic state in which an abnormality of cardiac function is responsible for the failure of the heart to pump blood at a rate commensurate with the requirements of the metabolizing tissues."[2] However, such a definition, although precise, is difficult to use in clinical practice. The definition of systolic heart failure that is used clinically is that it is "a syndrome which results from reduced left ventricular ejection fraction."[3] Systolic heart failure is also termed "heart failure with reduced ejection fraction" (HFREF). The pathophysiologic definition of diastolic heart failure is that "it is a condition resulting from an increased resistance to filling of one or both ventricles leading to symptoms of

Division of Cardiology, Department of Medicine, University of Iowa, Room/Bldg-E-314-4 GH, 200 Hawkins Drive, Iowa city, IA 52242-1081, USA
E-mail address: kanu-chatterjee@uiowa.edu

Med Clin N Am 96 (2012) 891–899
http://dx.doi.org/10.1016/j.mcna.2012.07.001
0025-7125/12/$ – see front matter Published by Elsevier Inc.

congestion due to an inappropriate shift of the diastolic-pressure volume relation (that is during the terminal phase of the cardiac cycle."[4]

The clinical definition of diastolic heart failure is that "it is a clinical syndrome characterized by the symptoms and signs of heart failure, a preserved left ventricular ejection fraction and abnormal diastolic function."[5] Diastolic heart failure is also termed "heart failure with preserved ejection fraction" (HFPEF). In this review, the terms systolic and diastolic heart failures are used instead of HFREF and HFPEF.

Pathophysiology

In systolic heart failure, the left ventricle is dilated and there is increase in both left ventricular end-diastolic and end-systolic volumes; but, as there is a greater increase in end-systolic than in end-diastolic volume, left ventricular ejection fraction is reduced. Ejection fraction is the ratio of left ventricular total stroke volume and its end-diastolic volume. Thus, when there is a disproportionate increase in end diastolic volume, ejection fraction may decline and the stroke volume may remain normal (**Fig. 1A**). Left ventricular stroke volume is the difference between end-diastolic and end-systolic volume. In some patients, when there is a disproportionate decrease in stroke volume, ejection fraction may decline despite normal left ventricular end-diastolic volume (see **Fig. 1B**).

There are substantial changes in the shape of the left ventricle. Normally, the left ventricle is ellipsoidal. In systolic heart failure, it becomes spherical. Changes to globular shape cause misalignment of the papillary muscles, chordate, and mitral valve leaflets, which is associated with mitral regurgitation. Mitral regurgitation causes further increase in left ventricular volumes and progressive remodeling.

In systolic heart failure, the left ventricular wall thickness remains unchanged or may decrease. The normal or decreased left ventricular wall thickness along with an increase in ventricular volumes is associated with increased wall stress (**Fig. 2**). There is an inverse relationship between wall stress and ejection fraction. The higher the wall stress, the lower is the ejection fraction. Thus, in patients with systolic heart failure, an increase in wall stress contributes to decreased ejection fraction. The major mechanism of reduced ejection fraction, however, is decreased contractility. The morphologic and functional changes in systolic heart failure are summarized in **Table 1**.

Left ventricular "Starling" function is depressed in patients with systolic heart failure. Ventricular "Starling" function is the relationship between its stroke volume

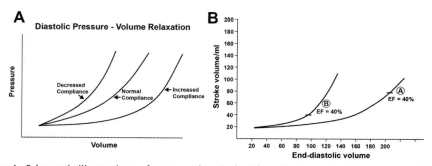

Fig. 1. Schematic illustrations of pressure (*vertical axis*) and volume (*horizontal axis*). When there is a disproportionate increase in end-diastolic volume, ejection fraction can be reduced with normal stroke volume (*A*). Ejection fraction may decrease to the same extent when there is a disproportionate decrease in stroke volume with normal end-diastolic volume (*B*).

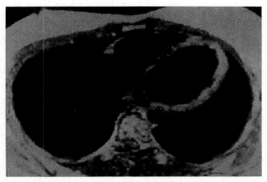

Fig. 2. Cardiac magnetic resonance image of a patient with systolic heart failure illustrating normal wall thickness and globular shape of the left ventricle.

and end-diastolic volume. In clinical practice, pulmonary capillary wedge pressure is used to represent left ventricular end-diastolic volume. In systolic heart failure, increased pulmonary capillary wedge pressure with reduced or normal stroke volume indicates depressed left ventricular "Starling" function (**Fig. 3**).

In systolic heart failure, left ventricular mass is increased, which can be measured by transthoracic echocardiography. Cardiac magnetic resonance imaging, however, is a more precise technique to measure left ventricular mass (see **Fig. 2**; see **Table 1**). Increased left ventricular mass is a result of left ventricular hypertrophy. Left ventricular mass cannot be detected by electrocardiography. The left ventricular cavity size is increased, which can also be detected by both echocardiography and cardiac magnetic resonance imaging. In systolic heart failure, left ventricular cavity size is markedly increased and the cavity/mass ratio is increased.

In patients with systolic heart failure, progressive left ventricular dilatation may occur, particularly in patients treated inadequately with pharmacotherapy of proven benefit. The angiotensin inhibitors, beta blockers, and aldosterone antagonists can attenuate progressive left ventricular dilatation and remodeling. Progressive ventricular dilatation is associated with worsening heart failure and poor prognosis.

In systolic heart failure, there are also substantial changes in the architecture of the extracellular matrix. The collagen fibrils are disrupted and disorganized. The collagen fibrils are thinner than normal.[6] Myocardial collagen volume and fibrosis increase in systolic heart failure. Circulating levels of procollagen are increased, which suggests abnormal collagen metabolism.[7]

Table 1 LV Mass volumes and EF in heart failure		
	Normals	**DCM**
LV mass	79.5 ± 7.6	152.5 ± 31.1
LVEDV	62.3 ± 7.3	116.8 ± 28.4
LVESV	21.7 ± 3.9	71.6 ± 23.9
LVEF	65.1 ± 3.6	35.1 ± 2.4
Wall stress	43.0 ± 10.7	91.2 ± 20.2

Abbreviations: DCM, dilated cardiomyopathy; EDV, end-diastolic volume; ESV, end-systolic volume; LV, left ventricular; LVEF, left ventricular ejection fraction.

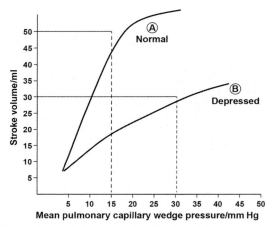

Fig. 3. Schematic illustration of left ventricular "Starling" function relating stroke volume (*vertical axis*) and pulmonary capillary wedge pressure (*horizontal axis*). In systolic heart failure, the ventricular function curve shifts downward and to the right. In diastolic heart failure, there is no shift of the ventricular function curve.

Neurohormonal Changes

Neurohormonal activation is a major pathophysiologic mechanism for ventricular remodeling and progression of heart failure in systolic heart failure.[8,9] There are increased levels of circulating catecholamines, such as norepinephrine and dopamine. There is also evidence for increased central nervous system–mediated activation of the sympathetic nervous system. The muscle sympathetic nerve activity is substantially increased in patients with systolic heart failure. The renin-angiotensin-aldosterone system is activated, as is evident from increased levels of plasma renin, angiotensin, and aldosterone. Angiotensin produces its deleterious effects by activation of angiotensin receptor subtype 1 receptors. There is vasoconstriction, and smooth muscle and myocyte hypertrophy. It also induces proinflammatory, mitogenic, and prothrombotic effects. Levels of vasopressins, endothelins, and cytokines, such as tumor necrosis factor-alpha, are also elevated. These neurohormones also induce vasoconstriction, and increase systemic vascular resistance, which is associated with deterioration in left ventricular systolic function. These neurohormones also exert proinflammatory, mitogenic, and prothrombotic effects. Aldosterone promotes collagen synthesis and fibrosis.

There is concurrent activation of vasodilatory, natriuretic, antimitogenic, and antithrombotic neurohormones. The levels of natriuretic peptides, such as B-type natriuretic peptide (BNP), nitric oxide, endothelium-derived relaxing factor, and prostacyclins are increased. It has been postulated that if the balance between these 2 systems is maintained, ventricular remodeling can be attenuated; however, progressive ventricular remodeling continues if there is an excessive activation of adrenergic and renin-angiotensin-aldosterone systems.

Hemodynamic Changes

The hemodynamic changes in systolic heart failure are characterized by an increase in pulmonary venous pressure secondary to increased left ventricular diastolic volumes. There is a passive increase in pulmonary artery pressure, which increases resistance to right ventricular emptying. As a result, right ventricular function deteriorates, which is clinically manifested by elevated jugular venous pressure (**Fig. 4**) and dependent

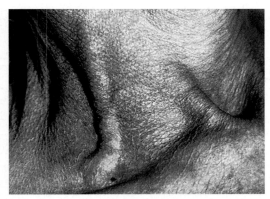

Fig. 4. Jugular venous distension in patients with heart failure is illustrated. Both external and internal jugular veins are distended owing to increased systemic venous pressure.

edema. With chronic elevation of pulmonary venous pressure, there is also an increase in pulmonary vascular resistance, which further increases right ventricular afterload. There may be a decrease in both right and left ventricular stroke volume, which is associated with signs and symptoms of low cardiac output. Left ventricular stroke volume decreases not only because of deceased contractility and increased afterload, but also because of decreased filling resulting from decreased right ventricular stroke volume, which contributes to left ventricular preload.

Mechanical dyssynchrony contributes to deranged hemodynamics in systolic heart failure. Mechanical dyssynchrony, in presence or absence of electrical dyssynchrony, is observed in approximately 30% to 40% of patients with systolic heart failure. When mechanical dyssynchrony is present, contraction and relaxation of the lateral wall occurs earlier than that of the interventricular septum. The mechanical dyssynchrony, although most frequently observed in patients with left bundle branch block, and with QRS duration of 140 ms or greater, it can be observed in patients with a narrow QRS complex. However, resynchronization therapy is not effective in patients with a narrow QRS complexes.

The mechanical dyssynchrony may be associated with decreased stroke volume and cardiac output without a significant change in ventricular volumes. The mechanical dyssynchrony is an important cause of secondary mitral regurgitation in systolic heart failure.

Diastolic Heart Failure

Morphologic changes

In diastolic heart failure, left ventricular cavity size remains normal or can be decreased. Left ventricular end-diastolic volume is normal or less than normal. The end-systolic volume is also decreased, but the magnitude of decrease in end-systolic volume is proportionately greater than that of end-diastolic volume. Thus, left ventricular ejection fraction remains normal. The left ventricular wall thickness is substantially increased in patients with diastolic heart failure. Left ventricular mass is increased in patients with diastolic heart failure. As the cavity size remains normal, the cavity/mass ratio is decreased (**Table 2**).

Reduced cavity size and increased wall thickness are associated with decreased left ventricular wall stress. Decreased wall stress is the predominant mechanism for

Table 2
Systolic versus diastolic heart failure

	SHF	DHF
EDV	Increased	Unchanged or decreased
ESV	Increased	Unchanged or decreased
LVEF	Decreased	Preserved
LV mass	Increased	Increased
LV wall thickness	Unchanged	Increased
LV wall stress	Increased	Decreased

Abbreviations: DHF, diastolic heart failure; EDV, end-diastolic volume; ESV, end-systolic volume; LV, left ventricle; LVEF, left ventricular ejection fraction; SHF, systolic heart failure.

maintaining normal ejection fraction in patients with diastolic heart failure. In patients with a symptomatic diastolic heart, left ventricular volumes remain unchanged and there is no ventricular dilatation. There is, however, increased wall stiffness, which is associated with worsening hemodynamics and symptoms of heart failure.[10,11]

The changes in myocytes in diastolic heart failure are characterized by an increase in its thickness without any change in its length. There is an increase in the thickness of the collagen bundles surrounding the myocytes but the collagen volumes remain unchanged.[6]

Neurohormonal Changes

The neurohormonal changes in systolic and diastolic heart failure are similar.[12] There is an increase in plasma levels of catecholamines. There is also increased activation of the rennin-angiotensin and aldosterone system. Concurrently there is activation of vasodilatory, antimitogenic, and natriuretic peptides. The circulating levels of pro-BNP and BNP are increased in diastolic heart failure.

Although neurohormonal changes in systolic and diastolic heart failure are similar, the effects on ventricular remodeling appear different. In systolic heart failure, there is dilatation of the left ventricle with an increase in end-diastolic and end-systolic volumes. In diastolic heart failure, the ventricular size remains unchanged without an increase in end-diastolic and end-systolic volumes.

Functional Derangements

The principal functional abnormality in diastolic heart failure is increased left ventricular wall stiffness and decreased compliance. The pressure volume relation is shifted upward and to the left. For any given increase in left ventricular volume, there is a disproportionate increase in left ventricular diastolic pressure. The left ventricular contractile function and ejection fraction remain normal; however, some echocardiographic parameters of contractile function may be decreased.

Hemodynamic Changes

Decreased left ventricular compliance is associated with increased left ventricular diastolic pressure. Concurrently, left atrial and pulmonary venous pressures increase with symptoms and signs of pulmonary venous congestion. When there is a marked decrease in left ventricular compliance, left ventricular filling is restricted. As a result, stroke volume and cardiac output decrease with signs and symptoms of low cardiac output. Pulmonary venous hypertension is associated with an obligatory increase in pulmonary artery pressure. Pulmonary artery pressure is right ventricular afterload and increased pulmonary artery pressure (increased afterload) is associated with right ventricular failure associated with increased right ventricular diastolic and right atrial pressures. Thus, signs and symptoms of systemic venous hypertension, such as peripheral edema, occur despite normal left ventricular ejection fraction.

Diagnosis of Systolic and Diastolic Heart Failure

The symptoms and signs are similar in both systolic and diastolic heart failure. Exertional dyspnea, paroxysmal nocturnal dyspnea, and orthopnea are observed in both types of heart failure. Typical angina is uncommon in patients with systolic or diastolic heart failure. Signs of pulmonary venous congestion, such as pulmonary rales, and of systemic venous congestion, such as elevated jugular venous pressure and lower extremity edema, can be present in both systolic and diastolic heart failure.

Chest radiograph may reveal cardiomegaly and radiologic findings of hemodynamic pulmonary edema (**Fig. 5**). For establishing the diagnosis, however, a transthoracic echocardiography is essential. In patients with systolic heart failure, left ventricular ejection fraction is reduced to less than 45% and in diastolic heart failure, it is normally usually 50% or higher.

Therapeutic Strategies

There are substantial differences in the management of systolic and diastolic heart failure. The neurohormonal antagonists, which have been documented to decrease mortality and morbidity of patients with systolic heart failure, do not appear to be of benefit in patients with diastolic heart failure. Angiotensin inhibitors and adrenergic antagonists, which have been demonstrated as life-saving treatments in systolic heart failure, do not have any beneficial effects in diastolic heart failure. Aldosterone antagonists are useful in the management of patients with advanced systolic heart failure. It remains unclear whether such therapy will be of any benefit in patients with diastolic

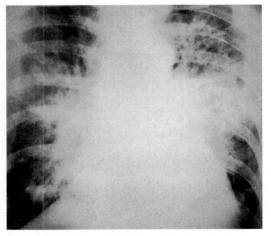

Fig. 5. A plain chest radiograph showing florid hemodynamic pulmonary edema. Pulmonary edema can occur in both systolic and diastolic heart failure.

heart failure. The combination therapy of hydralazine and isosorbide dinitrate produce substantial benefits in reducing mortality and morbidity of patients with systolic heart failure. Such treatment, however, is not effective in patients with diastolic heart failure. Exogenous BNP therapy is not effective in systolic or diastolic heart failure. Nonpharmacologic therapy, such as chronic resynchronization treatment, improves morbidity and mortality of patients with systolic heart failure. Such therapy, however, is not effective in diastolic heart failure. Phosphodiesterase-5 inhibitors may be effective in patients with diastolic heart failure, but they are not effective in patients with systolic heart failure. Forty-four patients with diastolic heat failure with ejection fraction higher than or equal to 50% and pulmonary artery systolic pressure higher than 40 mm Hg were randomized to receive either sildenafil 50 mg 3 times daily or placebo. At 6 and 12 months with sildenafil treatment, there was a significant reduction in mean pulmonary artery, right atrial, and mean pulmonary capillary wedge pressures. There was also a substantial reduction in pulmonary vascular resistance, but systemic vascular resistance and arterial pressure remained unchanged.[13] Thus, the beneficial effect of phosphodiesterase-5 inhibition was attributable to selective pulmonary vasodilatation in these patients. There was a concomitant symptomatic improvement and increased effort tolerance.

Diuretic therapies, however, are necessary to relieve congestive symptoms in both patients with systolic and diastolic heart failure. It should be appreciated that diuretic therapy may worsen the prognosis and cause deterioration of renal function. The treatment strategies in patients with systolic and diastolic heart failure are summarized in **Box 1**.

Box 1
Diastolic and systolic heart failure management strategies

Angiotensin-converting enzyme inhibitors and/or angiotensin receptor blockers:

- Decrease mortality and morbidity in systolic heart failure
- Decrease primarily morbidity in diastolic heart failure

Beta-blocker therapy:

- Decrease mortality and morbidity in systolic heart failure
- Unproven benefit in diastolic heart failure

Hydralazine-nitrate:

- Decrease mortality and morbidity in systolic heart failure
- Unproven benefit in diastolic heart failure

PDE-inhibition, beneficial in diastolic heart failure, is contraindicated in systolic heart failure.

Cardiac resynchronization and/or implantable cardioverter defibrillator:

Decrease mortality and morbidity in refractory systolic heart failure

Not indicated in diastolic heart failure

Implantable left ventricular assist device:

May improve short-term survival in selected patients with refractory systolic heart failure

Unproven benefit in diastolic heart failure

Cardiac transplantation:

May be of benefit in both systolic and diastolic heart failure

REFERENCES

1. Fishberg AM. Heart failure. Philadelphia: Lea & Febiger; 1937.
2. Braunwald E. Heart disease. In: Textbook of cardiovascular medicine. Philadelphia: WB Saunders; 1980.
3. Chatterjee K, Massie B. Systolic and diastolic heart failure: differences and similarities. J Card Fail 2007;13:569–76.
4. Brutsaert DL, Sys SU, Gillebert TC. Diastolic failure: pathophysiology and therapeutic implications. J Am Coll Cardiol 1993;22:318–25.
5. Zile MR, Brutsaert DL. New concepts in diastolic dysfunction and diastolic heart failure: part I: diagnosis, prognosis and measurements of diastolic function. Circulation 2002;105:1387–93.
6. Aurigema GP, Zile MR, Gaasch WH. Contractile behavior of the left ventricle in diastolic heart failure with emphasis on regional systolic function. Circulation 2006;113:296–304.
7. Rossi A, Cicoira M, Golia G, et al. Amino-terminal propeptide of type III procollagen is associated with restrictive mitral filling pattern in patients with dilated cardiomyopathy: a possible link between diastolic dysfunction and prognosis. Heart 2004;90:650–4.
8. Chatterjee K, DeMarco T, McGlothlin D. Remodeling in systolic heart failure—effects of neurohormonal modulators: basis for current pharmacotherapy. Cardiol Today 2005;9:270–7.
9. Aurigemma GP, Gaasch WH. Diastolic heart failure. N Engl J Med 2004;351:1097.
10. Handoko ML, van Heerebeek L, Bronzwaer JG, et al. Does diastolic heart failure evolve to systolic heart failure? Circulation 2006;114(Suppl II):816.
11. Van Heerbeek L, Borbely A, Niessen HW, et al. Myocardial structure and function differ in systolic and diastolic heart failure. Circulation 2006;113:1966–73.
12. Kitzman DW, Little WC, Brubaker PH, et al. Pathophysiological characterization of isolated diastolic heart failure in comparison to systolic heart failure. JAMA 2002; 288:2144–50.
13. Guazzi M, Vicenzi M, Arena R, et al. Pulmonary hypertension in heart failure with preserved ejection fraction. A target of phosphodiesterase-5 inhibition in a 1-year study. Circulation 2011;124:164–74.

The Appropriate Use of Biomarkers in Heart Failure

Punam Chowdhury, MD[a,b,*], Rajiv Choudhary, MD, MPH[c],
Alan Maisel, MD[a,b]

KEYWORDS

- Heart failure • Natriuretic peptides • Troponins • Cystasin-C • NGAL • KIM1 • ST2
- Galectin-3

KEY POINTS

- The activation of compensatory pathways and ongoing hemodynamic changes result in the release of biomarkers that can be monitored to chart disease progression and possibly target for therapy.
- We will review the biomarkers of heart failure that have been the focus of much discussion and research, including neurohormonal markers, particularly natriuretic peptides, cardiac injury markers, specifically troponins, inflammatory marker sST2, and matrix remodeling marker Galectin-3.
- In addition, we will discuss cardiorenal markers that have shown promise in improving risk stratification of patients with HF with worsening renal function, such as cystatin C, neutrophil gelatinase-associated lipocalin (NGAL), and kidney injury molecule-1 (KIM -1).

INTRODUCTION

Heart failure (HF) has a considerable morbidity, mortality, and economic burden in the United States. Per the Centers for Disease Control and Prevention data, in 2010, approximately 5.8 million people had HF in the United States and about 670,000 people are diagnosed with it each year.[1,2] HF was found to contribute to 282,754 deaths in 2006 and an estimated 1 in 5 patients with HF die within 1 year of diagnosis.[1,2] In addition, the estimated cost of HF for the United States was $39.2 billion in 2010.[1,2] The heavy burden of HF has made it the focus of research and much discussion. In conjunction with pharmacologic and device therapy, the new and growing focus is particularly on biomarkers for diagnostic, prognostic, and therapeutic use in managing HF.

Conflict of interest: Alan Maisel- consultant: Alere, Critical Diagnostics, EFG.
Research support: Alere, Abbott, Nanosphere, Brahms-thermofisher, Novartis.
[a] Department of Cardiology, San Diego Veterans Affairs Medical Center, 3350 La Jolla Village Drive, San Diego, CA 92101, USA; [b] University of California San Diego, 200 West Arbor Drive, San Diego, CA 92103, USA; [c] Capitol Health Medical Center, Trenton, NJ, USA
* Corresponding author. Department of Cardiology, San Diego Veterans Affairs Medical Center, 3350 La Jolla Village Drive, San Diego, CA 92101.
E-mail address: cPunam80@yahoo.com

HF is often seen secondary to inciting events, such as ischemic heart disease (IHD), hypertension, or arrhythmias, leading to LVSD (Left Ventricular Systolic Dysfunction) and poor cardiac output.[3,4] National heart failure registry databases have reported that most patients with HF have preserved left ventricular ejection fraction (LVEF), termed HFpEF.[5] The vicious cycle that ensues poor cardiac output is outlined in **Fig. 1**. Renal dysfunction is another entity plaguing patients with HF. In the acute setting, several factors, such as administration of nephrotoxic agents to overuse of diuretics, are responsible for worsening renal function in such patients, characterizing cardiorenal syndrome.[6] The activation of compensatory pathways and ongoing hemodynamic changes result in the release of biomarkers that can be monitored to chart disease progression and possibly target for therapy.[7]

There are several biomarkers of HF, and for a robust list please refer to **Box 1**. We review biomarkers that have been the focus of much discussion and research, including neurohormonal markers, particularly natriuretic peptides, cardiac injury markers, specifically troponins, inflammatory marker sST2, and matrix remodeling marker Galectin-3. In addition, we discuss cardiorenal markers that have shown promise in improving risk stratification of patients with HF with worsening renal function, such as cystatin C, neutrophil gelatinase-associated lipocalin (NGAL), and kidney injury molecule-1 (KIM-1).

NATRIURETIC PEPTIDES

Atrial natriuretic peptides (ANPs) are a family of hormones that all share a common 17 amino-acid ring structure and have natriuretic, diuretic, and/or kaliuretic properties.

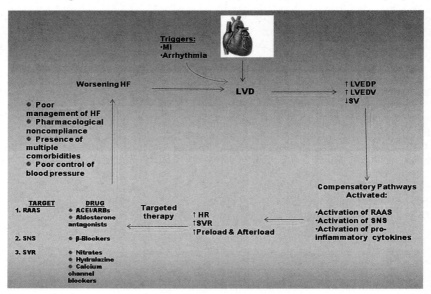

Fig. 1. Underlying pathophysiology seen in patients with HF. With poor cardiac output resulting from an initial triggering event, such as IHD, arrhythmias cause several hemodynamic changes and activate the neurohormonal, sympathetic, and inflammatory pathways. The following changes in heart rate and increase in vascular resistance are often seen as presenting signs on examination, especially in decompensated patients in addition to signs of fluid overload. Targeted therapy details pharmacologic management targeted at such ongoing dynamic changes so as to prevent exacerbation or worsening of symptoms. *Abbreviations:* HR, heart rate; LVEDP, left ventricular end-diastolic pressure; LVEDV, left ventricular end-diastolic volume; RAAS, renin-angiotensin-aldosterone system; SNS, sympathetic nervous system; SV, stroke volume; SVR, systemic vascular resistance.

There are 3 major types of human NPs, including natriuretic peptide (ANP), brain natri-uretic peptide (BNP), and C-type natriuretic peptide (CNP).[7] ANP is predominantly secreted from the atria, whereas BNP is mainly produced and released as a response to the degrees of ventricular stretch and ventricular dilatation.[7] CNP is mainly secreted from endothelial cells and has a role in regional blood flood.[8] Wall stretch of the ventri-cles triggers the cleavage and release of BNP (active hormone 79–108 amino-acid structure) and NT-pro BNP (the inactive fragment 1–76 amino-acid structure) from precursor prohormone[8] and has been associated with HF severity and prognosis. NPs, namely BNP and N-terminal-proBNP (NT-proBNP) have particularly shown diag-nostic, prognostic, and therapeutic value in patients with HF.

Diagnostic Value of NPs

In the Breathing Not Properly study, it was shown that at 100 pg/mL, BNP had a sensi-tivity of 90% and specificity of 73% of diagnosing HF in patients presenting to the emergency room.[9] It showed that BNP independently had better predictive value in diagnosing HF compared with the National Health and Nutrition Examination Survey and the Framingham criteria for diagnosing HF.[9] In the N-terminal Pro-BNP Investiga-tion of Dyspnea in the Emergency department (PRIDE) study, NT-proBNP values higher than 450 pg/mL for patients younger than 50 years of age and higher than 900 pg/mL for patients 50 years and older were highly sensitive and specific for the diagnosis of acute congestive HF (CHF) ($P<.001$) in initial presentation to the emer-gency room (ER) for dyspnea. NT-proBNP lower than 300 pg/mL was highly useful in ruling out CHF with a negative predictive value of 99%.[10] Studies have further shown that using NP for initial diagnosis and then therapy guidance has had a positive outcome compared with conventional therapy. Mueller and colleagues[11] had patients in the ER who presented with dyspnea randomly assigned to either a group involving the measurement of BNP levels with the use of a rapid bedside assay or to a group in which patients were assessed in a standard manner. The BNP level group had lower hospitalizations when compared with the control group (75% vs 85%, $P = .008$). Moreover, the BNP group had shorter hospital stay with lower median time to discharge (8 days vs 11 days, $P = .001$) compared with the control group. The BNP-level group also showed lower mean cost of treatment than standard care with $5410 (95% confidence interval [CI], $4516 to $6304) in the B-type NP group, versus $7264 (95% CI, $6301 to $8227) in the standard group ($P = .006$).

Prognostic Value of NPs

The Italian Research Emergency Department (RED) study showed that in acute decompensated HF, reducing BNP levels more than 46% at hospital discharge compared with the admission levels along with a BNP absolute value lower than 300 pg/mL had a powerful negative predictive value for future cardiovascular events.[12] Likewise, Doust and colleagues[13] did a systematic review of several studies that used BNP to estimate event rates in patients with HF and those who used BNP to estimate event rates in asymptomatic patients. They found that in patients with HF, each 100-pg/mL increase was associated with a 35% increase in the relative risk of death.

NP Therapy–Guided Treatment

Identifying patients with HF at increased risk of mortality and morbidity and tailoring treatment accordingly has been a daunting task. In an algorithm for NP-guided treat-ment for patients, the core of the algorithm signifies the percent reduction in NP levels to either intensify ongoing HF therapy or to discharge the patient so as to prevent unnecessary overuse of drugs. Studies thus far delving in the area of NP guided therapy

Box 1
Biomarkers of heart failure: suggested laboratory biomarkers for heart failure

Neurohormones

Natriuretic peptides (ANP, BNP, CNP, and related peptides) (1, 2, 3, 4, 5, 6)

Markers of rennin-angiotensin-aldosterone system activity (5)

Catecholamines (5)

Endothelins (5)

Chromogranin A and B (3)

Arginine vasopressin and copeptin (5)

Adrenomedullin (5)

Cortisol (5)

Leptin (5)

Adiponectin (1, 5)

Resistin (5)

Cardiac injury (necrosis, apoptosis) markers

Cardiac troponins (cTnI and cTnT) (1, 2, 4, 5)

Heart-type fatty acid binding protein (H-FABP) (5)

Fas (APO-1) (5)

Matrix remodeling, endothelial dysfunction, and inflammatory markers

Matrix metalloproteinases (MMPs) and MMP tissue inhibitors (4, 5)

Collagen propeptides (5)

Propeptide procollagen type I and procollagen type III (5)

Adhesion molecules (ICAM, selectin-P) (5)

C-reactive protein (1, 4, 5)

Cytokines and related receptors (interleukins: IL-1, IL-2, IL-6, IL-8, IL-18, TNF-α; osteoprotegerin; ST2; growth differentiation factor 15) (1, 4, 5)

Osteopontin (5)

Galectin 3 (5)

Pentraxin 3 (5)

Oxidative stress markers

Oxidized low-density lipoproteins (5)

Myeloperoxidase (5)

Urinary biopyrrins (5)

Isoprostanes (5)

Plasma malondialdehyde (3)

Serum uric acid (5)

Gamma-glutamyl transferasis (5)

Hormonal and other markers of cachexia

Alterations of hypophysial-adrenal axis (4, 5)

Tri-iodothyronine (4, 5)

IGF-1 and GH (5)

Cholesterol (4, 5)

Genetic tests

Genetic analysis of cardiomyopathies (monogenic and nonmonogenic forms of dilated cardiomyopathy) (1)

Genetic determinants of drug response (angiotensin-converting enzyme [ACE]-inhibition and beta-blockade) (ACE insertion/deletion—ACE II/DD-; Arg389Gly Beta-1 adrenergic receptor; Ser49Gly Beta-1 adrenergic receptor; Gln27Glu Beta-2 adrenergic receptor; Cytochrome P450 2D6 (CYP2D6) (6)

Comorbidities

Hemoglobin (5)

Creatinine and estimates of glomerular filtration rate (5)

Biomarkers are identified (see numbers within brackets) according to the classification proposed in Box 1: 1, Antecedent index (risk factor); 2, Screening index; 3, Diagnostic index; 4, Staging index; 5, Prognostic index; 6, Therapeutic monitoring index.

Data from Emdin M, Vittorini S, Passino C, Clerico A. Old and new biomarkers of heart failure. Eur J Heart Fail. 2009 Apr;11(4):331–5.

have been few and controversial. In the BATTLESCARRED (NT-proBNP-Assisted Treatment To Lessen Serial Cardiac Readmissions and Death) study, 364 patients with HF were randomized to therapy guided by NT-proBNP levels or by intensive clinical management or to a usual care group. The data showed that the 1-year mortality was similar in the hormone (9.1%) and clinically guided (9.1%) groups but lower in the usual care group (18.9%; $P = .03$). Three-year mortality was improved in patients 75 years or younger receiving hormone-guided therapy (15.5%) versus patients who were either in the clinically managed treatment (30.9%; $P = .048$) or usual care treatment group (31.3%; $P = .021$).[14] Similar findings were found in interim data from the PROTECT study, which showed improved mortality in the NT-pro BNP therapy–guided group as well[15]; however, some studies show equivocal results for therapy guided to NP. Interestingly, the study by Eurlings and colleagues[16] demonstrated that although HF therapy guided by individualized NP level helped identify those at increased risk, it failed to improve mortality and morbidity, possibly because of inadequacies in current standard HF therapy. Despite several limitations in the study design, it helped pave the way for future studies attempting to tailor treatment according to individualized targets.[16]

Evidently, bio-monitoring of NP levels may help identify those at high risk and possibly lower mortality in the younger population; perhaps future research may benefit from testing composite end points with longer follow-ups in a more heterogeneous population.

CARDIAC TROPONINS

The next biomarker that has been well studied is high-sensitivity cardiac troponin and is of significant diagnostic and prognostic use in patients with HF. Troponins are composed of 3 proteins (Troponin I, T, and C) that regulate calcium channel–mediated actin and myosin-induced muscle contraction.[17] Troponin I and T exist in cardiac and skeletal muscle and bioassays are used to measure those unique to cardiac tissue that are released during cardiac cell necrosis.[17] More recently, with the development of high-sensitivity cardiac troponin (hs-cTn), it is now possible to accurately measure troponin concentrations ≤99% of the healthy population and this makes it possible to detect previously undetectable levels.[18]

Diagnostic and Prognostic Utility of Troponin T and Troponin I

Metra and colleagues[19,20] conducted a study with 198 patients with acute decompensated HF with no signs of acute coronary syndrome and serially measured high-sensitivity (hs) cardiac troponin T (cTnT) at admission, 6 hours, and 12 hours. In the follow-up of these patients at a median of 247 days (interquartile range [IQR] 96–480 days), cTnT release was associated with an independent predictor of all-cause death and cardiovascular readmission rate. Increased cTnT levels were also associated with a higher rate of all-cause deaths. Kusumoto and colleagues[21] found significant correlation between hs-cTnT and cardiac dysfunction in patients with HF evaluated by echocardiography and BNP. Using multiple variable regression analysis, loghs-hs-cTnT independently correlated with LVEF, E/E', RV Tei index, and estimated glomerular filtration rate (eGFR). Loghs-hs-cTnT significantly correlated with logBNP ($R = 0.567$, $P<.0001$) or logNT-proBNP ($R = 0.647$, $P<.0001$). Masson and colleagues[22] analyzed 5284 patients with chronic HF from 2 independent randomized clinical trials, Val-HeFT (n = 4053) and GISSI-HF trial (n = 1231). They found hs-cTnT concentrations were associated with all-cause mortality; incidence rates were 8.19 (7.51–8.88) and 6.79 (5.98–7.61) per 100 person-years in Val-HeFT (Valsartan Heart Failure Trial) and GISSI-HF (Gruppo Italiano per lo Studio della Sopravvivenza nell'Insufficienza Cardiaca-Heart Failure), respectively, and hazard ratio (HR) 1.59 (95% confidence interval [CI], 1.39–1.82) and 1.88 (95% CI,1.50–2.35) after adjustment for conventional risk factors, baseline levels of hs-cTnT, and N-terminal pro-BNP. Further, Masson and colleagues[22] found that changes in hs-cTnT only had limited prognostic value in serial measurements specifically in fatal outcomes only.

Review of studies revealed that high-sensitivity cardiac Troponin I (hs-cTnI) has significant diagnostic and prognostic value. In a study by Arenja and colleagues,[23] hs-cTnI was measured in 667 patients who presented with dyspnea. Three classifications were used for hs-cTnI levels: below the limit of detection (<0.01 μg L[−1]), detectable but within the normal range (0.01–0.027 μg L[−1]), and increased levels (≥0.028 μg L[−1], ≥99th percentile). During the in-patient stay, mortality increased in patients with acute HF in correlation to increase in hs-cTnI in the 3 levels of 2%, 5%, and 14%, $P<.001$, respectively. One-year mortality also correlated with increasing hs-cTnI in the 3 levels of 21%, 33%, and 47%, $P<.001$, respectively. In addition, after adjustment of other risk factors, hs-cTnI remained an independent predictor of 1-year mortality (adjusted odds ratio [OR] 1.03 for each increase of 0.1 μg L[−1], 95% CI 1.02–1.05, $P<.001$) . Of note, the diagnostic accuracy of hs-cTnI for the diagnosis of acute HF as quantified by the area under the receiver operating characteristic curve was 0.78 (95% CI, 0.75–0.82).[23] Similarly, Kawahara and colleagues[24] found that in patients with nonischemic CHF, serial hs-cTnI at baseline, 6 months, and prospectively for about 4.25 years, the HR for mortality in patients with high hs-cTnI (≥0.03 ng/mL) and an increase in hs-cTnI (Δhs-cTnI ≥0 ng/mL) was 3.59 (95% CI 1.3–9.9, $P = .014$) versus those patients with high hs-cTnI (≥0.03 ng/mL) and a decrease in hs-cTnI (Δhs-cTnI <0 ng/mL) in serial markers. They also showed that in multivariate analysis, baseline hs-cTnI (≥0.03 ng/mL, $P = .0011$), as well as an increase in serial (6-month) cTnI (Δhs-cTnI ≥0 ng/mL, $P = .022$) were independent and important predictive biomarkers in nonischemic congestive HF.

BIOMARKER ST2

The third biomarker of focus is ST2. ST2 is an interleukin (IL)-1 receptor family member and exists in transmembrane form (ST2L) and soluble form (sST2).[25] IL-33 is the functional ligand for ST2, and the ligand of ST2L/IL-33 signals cardiac remodeling.[26] Studies have shown that sST2, which is a soluble decoy for IL-33, is increased in patients with HF and of particular value for prognostic value in patients with HF.[25,26]

Prognostic Utility of ST2

sST2 data include Pascual-Figal and colleagues'[27] study in hospitalized patients for acute decompensated HF. Admission hs-TnT, NT-proBNP, and sST2 levels were measured and patients were followed for about 2 years. It was found that sST2 (per 10 ng/mL, HR 1.09, 95% CI 1.04–1.13; $P<.001$), hs-TnT (per 0.1 ng/mL, HR 1.16, 95% CI 1.09–1.24; $P<.001$), and NT-proBNP (per 100 pg/mL, HR 1.01, 95% CI 1.003–1.01; $P<.001$) were each independently predictive of mortality. The study showed that if the levels of each of these biomarkers were below the mentioned cutoffs, then the mortality of the patients was 0% compared with 53% if all 3 biomarkers were elevated on follow-up.[27] The adjusted analysis showed that for each elevated marker, the risk of death tripled.[27] The prognostic nature of sST2 was also demonstrated by Januzzi and colleagues[28] in a study of acutely dyspneic patients presenting to the ER who were followed for 4 years. Of the biomarkers checked, several biomarkers were significant predictors of death, including sST2 (HR = 1.38; $P<.001$), along with log-transformed concentrations of hemoglobin (HR = 0.77; $P<.001$), and NT pro-BNP (HR = 1.19; $P<.001$). Manzano-Fernandez and colleagues[29] further showed that regardless of whether patients had decompensated HF with preserved ejection fraction (EF) or reduced EF (<50%), sST2 concentration is an independent predictor of mortality even though the concentration of sST2 was normally lower in those patients with preserved EF. In addition, Bayes-Genis and colleagues[30] showed that in the outpatient setting, sST2 improves risk stratification in patients with decompensated HF. They determined the sST2, NT-proBNP, and Framingham criteria of HF severity score for patients at baseline and 2 weeks, and followed the patients for 1 year for cardiac events. After variable adjustment, sST2 remained an independent predictor of risk (OR = 1.054; 95% CI, 1.01–1.09; $P = .017$). The optimum cutpoint for the sST2 ratio determined by receiver operating curve (ROC) analysis was 0.75. They also showed that 72% of patients with sST2 ratio greater than 0.75 and a baseline NT-proBNP level higher than 1000 ng/L had a cardiac event ($P = .018$) versus no cardiac events in patients below these cutoff values.[30] sST2 has shown significant promise in prognostic use in HF, especially when combined with other biomarkers like NPs, and there are very likely future studies to be published regarding this biomarker.

GALECTIN-3

The fourth biomarker discussed is Galectin-3. Progression of HF occurs when myocytes are replaced with tissue fibrosis or crosslinked collagen. A relatively new biomarker, Galectin-3 was found to be secreted by macrophages because of neurohormonal and mechanical stimuli, which in turn stimulate cells like fibroblasts, macrophages, and pericytes. The stimulus of these cells then leads to cell proliferation and procollagen I secretion that causes crosslinking collagen fibers and cardiac fibrosis.[31]

Progonostic Utility of Galectin-3

De Boer and colleagues[32] showed that in patients with HF, doubling of Galectin-3 levels, after correction for age, gender, BNP, eGFR, and diabetes, showed an HR of 1.38 (1.07–1.78; P = .015) for the primary outcome of all-cause mortality and HF hospitalization. The predictive value seemed to be stronger in patients with HF with preserved EF compared with those with decreased EF (P<.001). Combining plasma Galectin-3 and BNP levels increased prognostic value over either biomarker alone (ROC analysis, P<.05). Shah and colleagues[33] evaluated dyspneic patients with initial Galectin-3 levels and echocardiogram done during admission. Results showed elevated Galectin-3 levels was associated with tissue Doppler E/E(a) ratio, lower right ventricular (RV) fractional area change, higher RV systolic pressure, and more severe mitral or tricuspid regurgitation.[33] In a multivariate Cox regression model, Galectin-3 was a significant predictor of 4-year mortality independent of echocardiographic markers of risk.[33] The study further showed that patients with HF and Galectin-3 levels above the median value had a 63% mortality rate versus 37% mortality in those with levels below the median (P = .003).[33] A substudy of the CARE-HF (Cardiac Resynchronization in Heart Failure) trial conducted by Lopez-Andres and colleagues[34] showed serum levels of Galectin-3 higher than 30 ng/mL was associated with death (OR 2.98, 95% CI 1.43–6.22, P = .004) or HF-related hospitalization, along with left ventricular end-systolic volume higher than 200 mL (OR 3.42, 95% CI 1.65–7.10; P = .001).

CARDIORENAL BIOMARKERS

The last set of biomarkers we discuss are the cardiorenal biomarkers that have shown promise in patients with HF, specifically in those patients with renal impairment. It has been well recognized that patients with HF with renal dysfunction have poor prognosis.[8,35–37] The extent of dysfunction of each organ can be anywhere in a spectrum of severity and the renal disease can be mild to moderate, end-stage renal disease, or the patients may even have cardiorenal syndrome.

Cystatin C

Cystatin C is a novel endogenous marker of renal function of the family of cysteine proteinase inhibitors. Cystatin C moves freely across the glomerular membrane and is catabolized in the proximal tubules.[8] Cystatin C has been shown to be sensitive for detecting mild to moderate decrease of GFR, and has been shown to detect acute kidney injury 24 to 48 hours earlier than changes in creatinine.[8]

Prognostic utility of cystatin C

Cystatin C has proved superior to serum creatinine in detecting worsening renal function in patients with HF, as demonstrated by Damman and colleagues,[38] not to mention Cystatin C was of strong prognostic value (HR 2.27, 95% CI 1.12–4.63) within 24 months.[38] Lassus and colleagues[39] conducted a multicentered prospective study on 480 patients with acute HF that showed that Cystatin C, serum creatinine, and systolic blood pressure on admission along with age and gender, were independent prognostic risk factors. Further Cystatin C above median 1.30 mg/L was associated with the highest adjusted HR, 3.2 (95% CI 2.0–5.3), P<.0001, and combined use of NT-proBNP and cystatin C improved risk stratification. The study also demonstrated that at 12 months, patients with normal plasma creatinine with elevated cystatin C levels was associated with significantly higher mortality of 40.4% compared with 12.6% in patients with both markers within normal range, P<.0001.[39] Cystatin C therefore demonstrated substantial prognostic utility in HF even in the presence of normal kidney function. Gao and colleagues[40] demonstrated that in patients admitted with HF, elevated Cystatin C (1.63 ± 0.81 vs 0.91 ± 0.27 mg/L; $P<.01$) levels were associated with adverse outcomes (eg, cardiac death, heart transplantation, or progressive HF). In addition, Cystatin C, along with serum homocysteine and hs-C-reactive protein, were all independent predictors of adverse outcomes . Further, Manzano-Fernandez and colleagues[41] not only showed that the highest tertile of Cystatin C was an independent risk factor of adverse events in patients with HF compared with creatinine and the MDRD equation, they also showed that in a multimarker approach combining cardiac troponin T, N-terminal-proBNP, and Cystatin C improved risk stratification in an unselected cohort of patients with HF showing that patients with 2 (HR 2.37, 95% CI 1.10–5.71) or 3 (HR 3.64, 95% CI 1.55–8.56) elevated biomarkers had a higher risk for adverse events than patients with no elevated biomarkers ($P = .015$). The utility of Cystatin C is therefore not limited to renal disease but extends to cardiac disease, especially HF. With future studies expanding our knowledge on its use in patients with HF, Cystatin C demonstrates strong evidence of prognostic value in HF.

NGAL

The second cardiorenal biomarker that has received much attention is NGAL. NGAL or 24p3 and lipocalin -2, is member of the lipocalin superfamily of proteins.[8] It is a 25-kDa secretory glycoprotein that was initially identified in human neutrophil granule.[8] NGAL in serum and urine is an excellent measure of early acute renal injury with an area under the receiver operating characteristic curve of 0.90.[8,42] Rise in NGAL occurs at 24 to 48 hours, before the rise in creatinine, and in certain studies, serum NGAL was rapidly induced within 3 hours of tubule cell necrosis and apoptosis.[42,43]

Diagnostic and prognostic utility of NGAL

NGAL has also been shown to have significant prognostic value in patients with HF and renal disease. Aghel and colleagues[44] showed that in patients with acute decompensated HF, high admission serum NGAL levels were associated with higher likelihood of worsening renal failure (OR 1.92, 95% CI 1.23–3.12, $P = .004$). Also, patients with acute decompensated HF and NGAL of 140 ng/mL or higher had a 7.4-fold increased risk of developing worsening renal failure (sensitivity 86% and specificity of 54%).[44] Alvelos and colleagues[45] showed in that patients with acute HF, BNP and NGAL were independent predictors of the occurrence of both all-cause death and the combined end point. NGAL levels in the 75th percentile (>167.5 ng/mL) were associated with a 2.7-fold increase in the risk of death and a 2.9-fold increase in the risk of the first occurrence of hospitalization or death.[45] Further, in the GALLANT trial, Maisel and colleagues[46] showed that not only did increase in NGAL have higher rates of adverse events in patients with acute decompensated heart, they also showed that addition of discharge NGAL to BNP improved classification 10.3% in those with events and 19.5% in those without event ($P = .010$). Also, the study showed that patients with acute decompensated HF with elevated BNP and NGAL were at significant risk (HR 16.85, $P = .006$) along with patients with acute decompensated HF with low BNP and high NGAL (HR = 9.95, $P = .036$).[46] In the Rancho Bernado study, NGAL clearly showed independent cardiovascular risk participants without known cardiovascular disease during a mean time period of 11 years regardless of renal function. The results showed that NGAL was a significant predictor of cardiovascular disease mortality (HR 1.33, 95% CI 1.12–1.57), all-cause mortality (HR 1.19, 95% CI 1.07–1.32), and a combined cardiovascular end point (HR 1.26, 95% CI 1.10–1.45). The study also showed that NGAL adds incremental predictive value to NT-proBNP and C-reactive protein for cardiovascular mortality.[47,48]

KIM-1

The last cardiorenal biomarker we discuss is KIM-1, a type 1 transmembrane protein undetectable in the normal kidney but is expressed at high levels in human kidneys with de-differentiated proximal tubule epithelial cells after ischemic or toxic injury.[49] KIM-1 is cleaved from the surface of activated tubular cells and released into the urine by a metalloproteinase—a process regulated by the MAP kinase signaling pathways activated by cell stress.[50] Ichimura and colleagues[51] suggested that activated renal proximal tubular epithelial cells also phagocytose apoptotic cells using Kim-1 as a critical receptor.

Prognostic utility of KIM-1

Recent studies have shown that KIM-1 has significant prognostic value in HF, especially in those with renal disease. Jungbauer and colleagues[52] did a study on patients with chronic HF and found that urinary KIM-1 was significantly elevated in patients with HF compared with healthy controls (1100, IQR 620–1920 vs 550, IQR 320–740 ng/g urinary creatinine, $P<.001$). KIM-1 increased significantly with decreasing left ventricular function and severity of New York Heart Association class. Kidney injury molecule-1 along with N-acetyl-β-d-glucosaminidase were also predictors of all-cause mortality and the composite of all-cause mortality and re-hospitalization for HF (all $P<.05$). Similarly, Damman and colleagues[53] demonstrated that in patients with chronic HF, increase in markers of tubular damage, such as eGFR, urinary albumin, NAG, KIM-1, and NGAL, was associated with all-cause mortality and HF-related hospitalizations. Furthermore, in the presence of normal eGFR, elevated levels of KIM-1 and NGAL carried a poor prognosis.[53] KIM-1's prognostic benefit is marked in these studies discussed but data are limited and further studies are certainly needed for its clinical use. The other reason urinary KIM-1 is very exciting is because it is less invasive and does not require venipuncture for measurement.

SUMMARY

Cardiac biomarkers have recently been the center of attention, given their diagnostic, prognostic, and even therapeutic use in patients with HF. Natriuretic peptides and troponins have been extensively studied and used in HF and their value has been extensively discussed. sST2 and Galectin are also showing strong prognostic value in patients with HF and have been the focus of recent studies. HF in the presence of renal disease is common and has been a focus in recent studies because of the high mortality in these patients. Renal markers like Cystasin-C, NGAL, and KIM-1 have shown growing utility in HF. Their prognostic value is extremely promising and clinical use of these markers is being evaluated in current studies.

REFERENCES

1. CDC. Division for heart disease and stroke prevention. 2010. Available at: http://www.cdc.gov/dhdsp/data_statistics/fact_sheets/fs_heart_failure.htm. Accessed May 10, 2012.
2. Lloyd-Jones D, Adams RJ, Brown TM, et al. Heart disease and stroke statistics—2010 update. A report from the American Heart Association Statistics Committee and Stroke Statistics Subcommittee. Circulation 2010;121:e1–170.

3. De Luca L, Fonarrow GC, Kirkwood F, et al. Acute heart failure syndromes: clinical scenarios and pathophysiologic targets. Heart Fail Rev 2007;12:97–104.
4. Weintraub NL, Collins SP, Pang PS, et al. Acute heat failure syndromes: emergency department presentation, treatment, and disposition: current approaches and future aims. Circulation 2010;122:1975–96.
5. Fonarrow GC, Heywood JT, Heidenreich PA, et al. Temporal trends in clinical characteristics, treatments, and outcomes for heart failure hospitalizations, 2002 to 2004: findings from Acute Decompensated Heart Failure National Registry (ADHERE). Am Heart J 2007;153:1021–8.
6. Sarraf M, Masoumi A, Schrier RW. Cardiorenal syndrome in acute decompensated heart failure. Clin J Am Soc Nephrol 2009;4:2013–26. http://dx.doi.org/10.2215/CJN.03150509.
7. Pandit K, Mukhopadhyay P, Ghosh S, et al. Natriuretic peptides: diagnostic and therapeutic use. Indian J Endocrinol Metab 2011;15:S345–53.
8. Iwanaga Y, Miyazaki S. Heart failure, chronic kidney disease, and biomarkers—an integrated viewpoint. Circ J 2010;74:1274–82.
9. McCullough PA, Nowak RM, McCord J, et al. B-type natriuretic peptide and clinical judgment in emergency diagnosis of heart failure: analysis from Breathing Not Properly (BNP) Multinational Study. Circulation 2002;106:416–22.
10. Januzzi JL Jr, Camargo CA, Anwaruddin S, et al. The N-terminal Pro-BNP investigation of dyspnea in the emergency department (PRIDE) study. Am J Cardiol 2005;95:948–54.
11. Mueller C, Scholer A, Laule-Kilian K, et al. Use of B-type natriuretic peptide in the evaluation and management of acute dyspnea. N Engl J Med 2004;350:647–54.
12. Di Somma S, Magrini L, Pittoni V, et al. In-hospital percentage BNP reduction is highly predictive for adverse events in patients admitted for acute heart failure: the Italian RED study. Crit Care 2010;14:R116.
13. Doust JA, Pietrzak E, Dobson A, et al. How well does B-type natriuretic peptide predict death and cardiac events in patients with heart failure: systematic review. BMJ 2005;330:625–34.
14. Lainchbury JG, Troughton RW, Strangman KM, et al. N-terminal pro-B-type natriuretic peptide-guided treatment for chronic heart failure: results from the BATTLE-SCARRED (NT-proBNP-Assisted Treatment To Lessen Serial Cardiac Readmissions and Death) trial. J Am Coll Cardiol 2009;55:53–60.
15. Bhardwaj A, Rehman SU, Mohammed A, et al. Design and methods of the Pro-B Type Natriuretic Peptide Outpatient Tailored Chronic Heart Failure Therapy (PROTECT) Study. Am Heart J 2010;159:532–8.
16. Eurlings LW, van Pol Petra EJ, Kok WE, et al. Management of chronic heart failure guided by individual N-terminal pro-B-type natriuretic peptide targets. J Am Coll Cardiol 2010;56:2090–100.
17. Persson H, Erntell H, Eriksson B, et al. Improved pharmacological therapy of chronic heart failure in primary care: a randomized study of NT-proBNP guided management of heart failure—SIGNAL-HF (Swedish Intervention study–Guidelines and NT-proBNP AnaLysis in Heart Failure). Eur J Heart Fail 2010;12:1300–8.
18. Thomas J, Wang MD. Significance of circulating troponins in heart failure if these walls could talk. Circulation 2007;16:1217–20.
19. Metra M, Bettari L, Pagani F, et al. Troponin T levels in patients with acute heart failure: clinical and prognostic significance of their detection and release during hospitalization. Clin Res Cardiol 2012;101(8):663–72.
20. Venge P, Johnston N, Lindahl B, et al. Normal plasma levels of cardiac troponin I measured by the high-sensitivity cardiac troponin I access prototype assay and

the impact on the diagnosis of myocardial ischemia. J Am Coll Cardiol 2009;54: 1165–72.

21. Kusumoto A, Miyata M, Kubozono T, et al. Highly sensitive cardiac troponin T in heart failure: comparison with echocardiographic parameters and natriuretic peptides. J Cardiol 2012;59:202–8.

22. Masson S, Anand I, Favero C, et al, Valsartan Heart Failure Trial (Val-HeFT) and Gruppo Italiano per lo Studio della Sopravvivenza nell'Insufficienza Cardiaca–Heart Failure (GISSI-HF) Investigators. Serial measurement of cardiac troponin T using a highly sensitive assay in patients with chronic heart failure: data from 2 large randomized clinical trials. Circulation 2012;125:280–8.

23. Arenja N, Reichlin T, Drexler B, et al. Sensitive cardiac troponin in the diagnosis and risk stratification of acute heart failure. J Intern Med 2011. http://dx.doi.org/ 10.1111/j.1365-2796.2011.02469.x.

24. Kawahara C, Tsutamoto T, Sakai H, et al. Prognostic value of serial measurements of highly sensitive cardiac troponin I in stable outpatients with nonischemic chronic heart failure. Am Heart J 2011;162:639–45.

25. Bhardwaj A, Januzzi JL Jr. ST2: a novel biomarker for heart failure. Expert Rev Mol Diagn 2010;10:459–64.

26. Sanada S, Hakuno D, Higgins LJ, et al. IL-33 and ST2 comprise a critical biome-chanically induced and cardioprotective signaling system. J Clin Invest 2007; 117:1538–49.

27. Pascual-Figal DA, Manzano-Fernández S, Boronat M, et al. Soluble ST2, high-sensitivity troponin T- and N-terminal pro-B-type natriuretic peptide: complemen-tary role for risk stratification in acutely decompensated heart failure. Eur J Heart Fail 2011;13:718–25.

28. Januzzi JL Jr, Rehman S, Mueller T, et al. Importance of biomarkers for long-term mortality prediction in acutely dyspneic patients. Clin Chem 2010;56: 1814–21.

29. Manzano-Fernández S, Mueller T, Pascual-Figal D, et al. Usefulness of soluble concentrations of interleukin family member ST2 as predictor of mortality in patients with acutely decompensated heart failure relative to left ventricular ejec-tion fraction. Am J Cardiol 2011;107:259–67.

30. Bayes-Genis A, Pascual-Figal D, Januzzi JL, et al. Soluble ST2 monitoring provides additional risk stratification for outpatients with decompensated heart failure. Rev Esp Cardiol 2010;63:1171–8.

31. McCullough PA, Olobatoke A, Vanhecke TE. Galectin-3: a novel blood test for the evaluation and management of patients with heart failure. Rev Cardiovasc Med 2011;12:200–10.

32. de Boer RA, Lok DJ, Jaarsma T, et al. Predictive value of plasma galectin-3 levels in heart failure with reduced and preserved ejection fraction. Ann Med 2011;43: 60–8.

33. Shah RV, Chen-Tournoux AA, Picard MH, et al. Galectin-3, cardiac structure and function, and long-term mortality in patients with acutely decompensated heart failure. Eur J Heart Fail 2010;12:826–32.

34. Lopez-Andrès N, Rossignol P, Iraqi W, et al. Association of galectin-3 and fibrosis markers with long-term cardiovascular outcomes in patients with heart failure, left ventricular dysfunction, and dyssynchrony: insights from the CARE-HF (Cardiac Resynchronization in Heart Failure) trial. Eur J Heart Fail 2012;14:74–81.

35. Klein L, Massie BM, Leimberger JD, et al, OPTIME-CHF Investigators. Admission or changes in renal function during hospitalization for worsening heart failure predict postdischarge survival: results from the Outcomes of a Prospective Trial

of Intravenous Milrinone for Exacerbations of Chronic Heart Failure (OPTIME-CHF). Circ Heart Fail 2008;1:25–33.

36. Gottlieb SS, Abraham W, Butler J, et al. The prognostic importance of different definitions of worsening renal function in congestive heart failure. J Card Fail 2002;8:136–41.

37. Damman K, Voors AA, Hilldge HL, et al, CIBIS-2 Investigators, Committees. Congestion in chronic systolic heart failure is related to renal dysfunction and increased mortality. Eur J Heart Fail 2010;12:974–82.

38. Damman K, van der Harst P, Smilde TD, et al. Use of cystatin C levels in estimating renal function and prognosis in patients with chronic systolic heart failure. Heart 2012;98:319–24.

39. Lassus J, Harjola VP, Sund R, et al. For the FINN-AKVA Study group. Prognostic value of cystatin C in acute heart failure in relation to other markers of renal function and NT-proBNP. Eur Heart J 2007;28:1841–7.

40. Gao C, Zhong L, Gao Y, et al. Cystatin C levels are associated with the prognosis of systolic heart failure patients. Arch Cardiovasc Dis 2011;104:565–71.

41. Manzano-Fernández S, Boronat-Garcia M, Albaladejo-Otón MD, et al. Complementary prognostic value of cystatin C, N-terminal pro-B-type natriuretic peptide and cardiac troponin T in patients with acute heart failure. Am J Cardiol 2009;103: 1753–9.

42. Ronco C. N-GAL: diagnosing AKI as soon as possible. Crit Care 2007;11(6):173.

43. Mishra J, Mori K, Ma Q, et al. Neutrophil gelatinase-associated lipocalin: a novel early urinary biomarker for cisplatin nephrotoxicity. Am J Nephrol 2004;24:307–15.

44. Aghel A, Shrestha K, Mullens W, et al. Serum neutrophil gelatinase-associated lipocalin (NGAL) in predicting worsening renal function in acute decompensated heart failure. J Card Fail 2010;16:49–54.

45. Alvelos M, Lourenço P, Dias C, et al. Prognostic value of neutrophil gelatinase-associated lipocalin in acute heart failure. Int J Cardiol 2011. [Epub ahead of print].

46. Maisel AS, Mueller C, Fitzgerald R, et al. Prognostic utility of plasma neutrophil gelatinase-associated lipocalin in patients with acute heart failure: the NGAL EvaLuation Along with B-type NaTriuretic Peptide in acutely decompensated heart failure (GALLANT) trial. Eur J Heart Fail 2011;13:846–51.

47. Daniels LB, Barrett-Connor E, Clopton P, et al. Plasma neutrophil gelatinase-associated lipocalin is independently associated with cardiovascular disease and mortality in community-dwelling older adults: the Rancho Bernardo Study. J Am Coll Cardiol 2012;59:1101–9.

48. Yndestad A, Landrø L, Ueland T, et al. Increased systemic and myocardial expression of neutrophil gelatinase-associated lipocalin in clinical and experimental heart failure. Eur Heart J 2009;30:1229–36.

49. Han WK, Alinani A, Wu CL, et al. Human kidney injury molecule-1 is a tissue and urinary tumor marker of renal cell carcinoma. J Am Soc Nephrol 2005;16:1126–34.

50. Rees AJ, Kain R. Kim-1/Tim-1: from biomarker to therapeutic target? Nephrol Dial Transplant 2008;23:3394–6.

51. Ichimura T, Asseldonk EJ, Humphreys BD, et al. Kidney injury molecule-1 is a phosphatidylserine receptor that confers a phagocytic phenotype on epithelial cells. J Clin Invest 2008;118:1657–68.

52. Jungbauer CG, Birner C, Jung B, et al. Kidney injury molecule-1 and N-acetyl-β-D-glucosaminidase in chronic heart failure: possible biomarkers of cardiorenal syndrome. Eur J Heart Fail 2011;13:1104–10.

53. Damman K, Masson S, Hillege HL, et al. Clinical outcome of renal tubular damage in chronic heart failure. Eur Heart J 2011;32:2705–12.

Evidence-Based Therapy for Heart Failure

Prakash C. Deedwania, MD[a,b],*, Enrique Carbajal, MD[a,b]

KEYWORDS

- Evidence-based therapy • Heart failure • Left ventricular dysfunction • Treatment

KEY POINTS

- Despite the overwhelming evidence of benefits with evidence-based therapy using renin-angiotensin-aldosterone system–blocking drugs and β-blocking agents in patients with heart failure and left ventricular systolic dysfunction, their application in clinical practice is less than ideal.
- These data clearly emphasize that considerable opportunity exists for the implementation of evidence-based therapy for patients with heart failure caused by left ventricular systolic dysfunction to improve the associated adverse prognosis.

Heart failure (HF) is a major public health problem, and it is associated with increased morbidity and mortality. As the US life expectancy increases and the population ages, the overall prevalence of HF continues to escalate. Furthermore, the improved survival of patients with myocardial infarction (MI) and that of those with longstanding hypertension also contribute to the increasing prevalence of HF. Although in general the prognosis of patients with HF is considered worse than that for patients with many cancers, the increasing use of effective selective therapies such as neurohormonal blockade in the treatment of patients with HF has led to considerable improvement in the prognosis. During the past several decades, some studies have demonstrated the benefits of treatment with vasodilators, angiotensin-converting enzyme inhibitors (ACEIs), angiotensin II receptor blockers (ARBs), β-blocking drugs, and aldosterone receptor blockers on clinical symptoms and morbidity and mortality in patients with HF. Based on the evidence available from these studies, various national and international guidelines established specific recommendations for the evidence-based therapy with these drugs in patients with HF.[1,2]

The authors have nothing to disclose.
[a] Division of Cardiology, Department of Medicine, Fresno Medical Education Program, University of California San Francisco, 2615 East Clinton Avenue, Fresno, CA 93703, USA; [b] VA Central California Health Care System, 2615 East Clinton Avenue, Fresno, CA 93703, USA
* Corresponding author. VA Central California Health Care System, Cardiology Division (IIIC), 2615 East Clinton Avenue, Fresno, CA 93703.
E-mail address: deed@fresno.ucsf.edu

Med Clin N Am 96 (2012) 915–931
http://dx.doi.org/10.1016/j.mcna.2012.07.010
0025-7125/12/$ – see front matter Published by Elsevier Inc.

The authors review the evidence supporting the use of various drugs in patients with HF secondary to left ventricular (LV) systolic dysfunction. Other articles in this issue provide an appropriate discussion of various other therapies in the setting of HF.

EVIDENCE-BASED THERAPY FOR HF

HF is a progressive disorder, and early identification of those at risk of developing signs and symptoms of HF is of paramount importance. The most recent American College of Cardiology/American Heart Association guidelines[1,2] (**Fig. 1**) have emphasized identification of individuals in stages A/B of HF with the goal of early intervention to prevent progressive deterioration in cardiac dysfunction and subsequent prevention of symptomatic HF. Stage A patients are those who have risk factors (eg, those with hypertension, diabetes mellitus [DM], obesity, coronary artery disease [CAD], etc) that can lead to cardiac dysfunction and the development of HF. The treatment of these underlying risk factors should attenuate or prevent the subsequent development of cardiac dysfunction. Stage B patients are those who have LV hypertrophy or impaired LV function but are still asymptomatic. Early intervention with appropriate therapy such as neurohormonal blockers should prevent the process of cardiac remodeling and further progression of LV dysfunction (eg, early use of ACEIs and β-blockers in the setting of acute MI). Stage C denotes patients in whom symptoms of HF have developed caused by underlying cardiac dysfunction and who require treatment of the symptoms of HF and to improve the related adverse prognosis. Stage D patients are those who have significantly advanced and/or refractory HF who are generally candidates for specialized advanced treatment strategies including mechanical support devices and inotropic drugs and consideration for cardiac transplantation and/or other surgical procedures.

The drugs that have proved to be unequivocally beneficial in prolonging survival and improving symptoms in patients with LV systolic dysfunction and HF are primarily those that block the heightened neuroendocrine activity and include renin-angiotensin-aldosterone system (RAAS)-blocking drugs (ACEIs, ARBs, aldosterone receptor–blocking agents) and β-blocking agents. In addition, the combination of vasodilating drugs (hydralazine–isosorbide dinitrate in fixed combination) is beneficial in African American patients receiving standard therapy for HF. Although diuretics are frequently used and necessary in patients with congestive symptoms with fluid accumulation, there is no evidence that the chronic use of diuretic therapy improves survival. Furthermore, appropriate therapy for myocardial ischemia when present in the setting of HF is also associated with improved clinical outcome. In the following section, the authors discuss the specific use of drug therapy primarily directed toward neurohormonal blockade of the RAAS and sympathoadrenergic system. As shown in **Fig. 2**, both the RAAS and the sympathetic nervous system (SNS) are activated with the onset of myocardial dysfunction in response to decreased cardiac output. Initially, such a response is adaptive and helps to maintain adequate tissue perfusion of vital organs by causing peripheral vasoconstriction. However, the continued chronic activation of the RAAS and SNS has significant adverse consequences (see **Fig. 2**) as a result of continued peripheral vasoconstriction, sodium retention, and hemodynamic alterations. In addition to activation of these systems, in particular, the RAAS has been shown to be associated with progressive myocardial remodeling, which leads to worsening LV dysfunction. Because of the critical role of these neuroendocrine alterations in the pathophysiology of LV dysfunction and HF, there has been continued effort during the past several decades to use agents that are effective in blocking the RAAS and SNS systems, not only to improve the symptoms but also to decrease

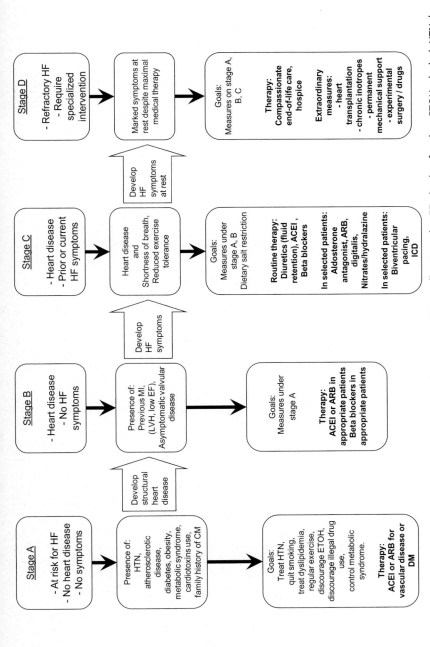

Fig. 1. Staging of heart failure and recommended therapy at various stages. CM, cardiomyopathy; EF, ejection fraction; ETOH, alcohol; HTN, hypertension; ICD, implantable cardioverter-defibrillator; LVH, left ventricular hypertrophy. (*Adapted from* Hunt SA, Abraham WT, Chin MH, et al. 2009 Focused update incorporated into the ACC/AHA 2005 guidelines for the diagnosis and management of heart failure in adults. Circulation 2009;119:e391–479.)

Neurohormonal Activation in Heart Failure

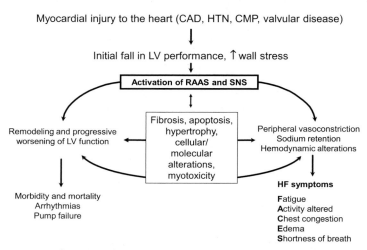

Fig. 2. Importance of RAAS and SNS activation in pathophysiologic process of heart failure. CMP, cardiomyopathy; HTN, hypertension; ↑, increased.

associated morbidity and mortality in patients with HF. The results of several studies have clearly demonstrated that the neurohormonal blockade of RAAS and SNS alleviates the symptoms of HF, improves clinical status and functional capacity, enhances sense of well-being, and reduces the associated morbidity and mortality in patients with HF.[3–10] Because of these well-demonstrated effects of RAAS-blocking drugs and β-blockers, treatment with these drugs has become part of the standard therapeutic armamentarium for all patients with HF. In the following sections, the authors discuss the rationale and the clinical application of these therapies in detail.

RAAS-BLOCKING DRUGS
ACEIs

ACEIs are the best-studied class of drugs in patients with HF, with multiple beneficial effects (**Fig. 3**). ACEIs should be prescribed for all patients with LV dysfunction and HF unless there is a contraindication for their use or the patient has a prior history of intolerance as a result of a significant adverse experience with these agents. Because of the well-demonstrated survival benefit even in those patients with asymptomatic LV dysfunction, treatment with ACEIs should not be delayed.

In patients with HF, the inhibition of ACE by ACEIs produces a moderate increase in cardiac output with a concomitant significant decrease in right ventricular and LV filling pressures, pulmonary and systemic vascular resistances, and mean arterial pressure, without increasing the heart rate. It is not established whether these effects of ACEI are caused entirely by the suppression of angiotensin II production, because ACE inhibition also enhances the production of bradykinin, which augments kinin-mediated prostaglandin production (see **Fig. 3**). ACEIs have other beneficial effects, including a reduction in the incidence of ventricular arrhythmias, decreased end-systolic and end-diastolic dimensions, and sustained improvements in symptoms, exercise duration, and quality of life.

ACEIs have been evaluated in several large, randomized controlled clinical trials of patients in various stages of HF, and these trials have universally shown a significant

RAAS In Heart Failure: ACEIs/ ARBs

Renin-Angiotensin System

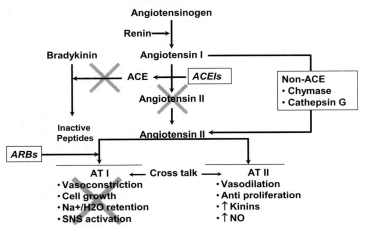

Fig. 3. Mechanism of action of ACEIs and ARBs. ATI-II, angiotensin II types I and II; NO, nitric oxide; ↑, increased.

reduction in mortality rates (**Table 1**).[3-9] All of these trials enrolled patients with reduced LV ejection fraction (LVEF <35%–40%) who were already receiving treatment with diuretics with or without digitalis and, in some cases, other vasodilating drugs. The aggregate results of these studies demonstrate a reduction in mortality of 20% to 25% in those treated with ACEIs compared with control groups.

Practical considerations regarding the use of ACEIs

Treatment with ACEIs should generally be initiated at low doses (**Table 2**) followed by gradual increments in dosage. Renal function and serum potassium levels should be assessed within 1 to 2 weeks of initiation of therapy and periodically thereafter,

Table 1
Summary of results from various studies showing effects of ACEIs on mortality

	Mortality		
Trial	ACEI, %	Controls	Relative risk (95% CI), %
HF			
CONSENSUS I	39	54	0.56 (0.34–0.91)
SOLVD (Treatment)	35	40	0.82 (0.70–0.97)
SOLVD (Prevention)	15	16	0.92 (0.79–1.08)
Post-MI			
SAVE (captopril)	20	25	0.81 (0.68–0.97)
AIRE (ramipril)	17	23	0.73 (0.60–0.89)
TRACE (trandolapril)	35	42	0.78 (0.67–0.91)
SMILE (zofenopril)	5	6.5	0.75 (0.40–1.11)

Abbreviations: AIRE, Acute Infarction Ramipril Efficacy; CI, confidence interval; CONSENSUS, COoperative North Scandinavian ENalapril SUrvival Study; SAVE, Survival And Ventricular Enlargement; SMILE, Survival of Myocardial Infarction Long-term Evaluation; SOLVD, Studies Of Left Ventricular Dysfunction; TRACE, TRAndolapril Cardiac Evaluation.

Table 2
List of evidence-based drugs and their dosage for HF

Drug	Initial Daily Dosage	Maximum Dosage
ACEIs		
Captopril	6.25 mg tid	50 mg tid
Enalapril	2.5 mg bid	10–20 mg bid
Fosinopril	5–10 mg qd	40 mg qd
Lisinopril	2.5–5 mg qd	20–40 mg qd
Perindopril	2 mg qd	8–16 mg qd
Quinapril	5 mg bid	20 mg bid
Ramipril	1.25–2.5 mg qd	10 mg qd
Trandolapril	1 mg qd	4 mg qd
ARBs		
Candesartan	4–8 mg qd	32 mg qd
Losartan	25–50 mg qd	50–100 mg qd
Valsartan	20–40 mg bid	160 mg bid
Aldosterone antagonists		
Spironolactone	12.5–25 mg qd	25 mg qd or bid
Eplerenone	25 mg qd	50 mg qd
β-Blockers		
Bisoprolol	1.25 mg qd	10 mg qd
Carvedilol	3.125 mg bid	25 mg bid; 50 mg bid if >85 kg
Metoprolol succinate extended release (CR/XL)	12.5–25 mg qd	200 mg qd
Hydralazine–isosorbide dinitrate in combination:		
With ACEI/ARB	Hydralazine 75 mg every 8 h plus isosorbide dinitrate 40 mg every 8 h	
Without ACEI/ARB	Hydralazine 50 mg every 6 h plus Isosorbide dinitrate 40 mg every 6 h	

Adapted from Hunt SA, Abraham WT, Chin MH, et al. 2009 Focused update incorporated into the ACC/AHA 2005 guidelines for the diagnosis and management of heart failure in adults: a report of the American College of Cardiology Foundation/American Heart Association Task Force on Practice Guidelines. Circulation 2009;119:e391–479.

particularly in patients with preexisting hypotension, hyponatremia, DM, or chronic kidney disease (estimated glomerular filtration rate <60 mL/min).

Differences among various ACEIs are primarily related to pharmacokinetic and hemodynamic properties. Captopril has the shortest duration of action, whereas enalapril, lisinopril, and other, newer ACEIs have a delayed onset of action and prolonged duration of hemodynamic effects. Many clinicians prefer to start treatment with captopril because of its shorter duration of action, especially in hospitalized patients who are ACEI naïve, to avoid the initial risk of hypotension, particularly in those patients who have low blood pressure (systolic blood pressure <80 mm Hg) or who are receiving high-dose diuretic therapy. However, in most stable patients, treatment with longer-acting agents starting at low doses can be initiated with careful monitoring. It is important to keep in mind that appropriate doses of diuretics need to be maintained in conjunction with the use of ACEIs because fluid retention can blunt the therapeutic effects and fluid depletion can potentiate the adverse effects of ACEIs.

The use of ACEIs is prohibited if the patient has previously experienced life-threatening adverse reactions (eg, angioedema, anuric renal failure). ACEIs should also be used with caution in patients who have low systolic blood pressure (<80 mm Hg), markedly increased serum creatinine levels (>3.0 mg/dL), bilateral renal artery stenosis, or elevated serum potassium levels (>5.5 mEq/L).

Another important issue concerns the optimal dose of ACEI in patients with HF. In most of the controlled clinical trials that were conducted to evaluate the survival benefit of treatment with ACEIs, the dose of ACEI was not determined by the patient's therapeutic response but rather was increased until the target dose was achieved. However, ACEIs are commonly prescribed in clinical practice at much lower doses that are similar to those recommended for initiation of therapy rather than maintenance of therapy (see **Table 2**). Clinicians should generally attempt to use the doses that have been shown to reduce the risk of mortality and other cardiovascular events in clinical trials. If the target doses of ACEIs cannot be used or are poorly tolerated, intermediate doses should be used. Furthermore, it is also important to note that although in some cases symptoms improve within a few days of starting treatment with ACEIs, in general, the clinical response to ACEI is delayed and requires several weeks, months, or longer. Even if symptoms do not improve, long-term treatment with ACEIs should be maintained to reduce the risk of death or hospitalization.

Many patients with HF who have previously received potassium supplementation in conjunction with diuretic therapy will not require such supplementation once they are on adequate doses of ACEIs. Therefore, it is important to monitor electrolytes and consider discontinuation of such supplementation at an appropriate time. Because it is well known that the use of nonsteroidal anti-inflammatory drugs (NSAIDs) can interfere with the favorable effects and enhance the adverse effects of ACEIs in patients with HF, their use should be avoided whenever possible. The concomitant use of aspirin has also been shown to be associated with decreased effects of ACEIs on cardiovascular morbidity and mortality. Despite these findings, when all the available data are considered together, the beneficial effects of ACEIs remain in patients both with and without aspirin therapy, and most physicians believe that when there is an indication for the use of aspirin, there is no harm in continuing it in conjunction with ACEI therapy.

Safety and adverse effects of ACEIs
Most of the adverse reactions of ACEIs are related to their principal pharmacologic actions: those related to angiotensin suppression, those related to kinin potentiation, and general reactions (eg, rash, taste disturbances).

Hypotension The most common adverse effects of ACEIs in patients with HF are hypotension and dizziness. Initially, blood pressure declines without symptoms in almost every patient treated with an ACEI. Therefore, a decrease in blood pressure should be a concern only if it is associated with syncope or other symptoms of cerebral hypoperfusion, postural symptoms, or worsening renal dysfunction. Significant hypotension, when present, is usually seen in the first few days of initiation of ACEI therapy or on an increase in the dosage. Some patients may be very sensitive to the hypotensive effects of ACEIs, particularly patients who are ACEI naïve and those who are dependent on the RAAS for blood pressure maintenance. This includes patients with hyponatremia or hypovolemia and those receiving high-dose diuretic therapy. The hypotension usually subsides with continued therapy and can be partly avoided by reducing the diuretic dosage or stopping it for few days ("diuretic holiday"). The patients considered to be at risk for hypotension should be monitored closely for the first 2 weeks of treatment. In some patients, a period of brief hospitalization and close observation during the initiation of ACEI therapy might be necessary.

Cough Cough is one of the most common reasons for the withdrawal of ACEIs. In general, the frequency of cough is between 5% and 10% in whites and has been reported to be higher in Asian populations. It is important to recognize that many patients with HF may have concomitant bronchitis, upper respiratory tract infection, or other conditions that may be the primary reason for their cough. Therefore, it is very important to establish that the cough is directly related to the use of ACEIs before discontinuing the ACEIs. It is also important to realize that worsening HF during decompensation can itself lead to cough caused by bronchial edema. It is therefore crucial to establish the link between the use of ACEIs and cough before considering the discontinuation of this lifesaving therapy in patients with HF. ACEI-induced cough generally occurs within the first few weeks or months of therapy, and it is usually nonproductive, generally persistent, and sometimes associated with an annoying "tickle" in the back of the throat. ACEI-induced cough generally disappears within 1 to 2 weeks of discontinuation of treatment and reappears with ACEI rechallenge. In several studies of ACEI-induced cough, it did not recur with rechallenge and was probably a coincidental finding. Unless the cough is severe and bothersome to the patient, clinicians should encourage patients to continue taking these drugs because of the well-demonstrated benefit on cardiovascular morbidity and mortality.

Renal dysfunction Because of the reduced renal perfusion in patients with HF, glomerular filtration rate is critically dependent on angiotensin-mediated efferent arteriolar vasoconstriction. Therefore, ACEIs might cause functional renal insufficiency by reducing the levels of angiotensin II. The risk of renal dysfunction secondary to ACEI use is greatest in those patients who are dependent on the renin-angiotensin system (RAS) for support of renal homeostasis. However, an increase in serum creatinine (eg, >0.3 mg/dL) is generally observed in 15% to 30% of patients with severe HF who are treated with ACEIs and in about 5% to 15% with mild to moderate HF. In most cases, this decline in renal function seems to be of little clinical significance. The risks are substantially greater if patient is taking NSAIDs or has baseline chronic kidney disease and/or bilateral renal artery stenoses. In most cases, however, renal function usually returns to baseline or stabilizes at a new steady state despite continued treatment with the ACEI. Renal function usually improves after reduction in dose of concomitantly administered diuretic, and thus these patients can generally be managed without the need to withdraw treatment with an ACEI. However, when clinically indicated, discontinuing treatment or decreasing the dose of the ACEI will also rapidly resolve the renal dysfunction. In major clinical trials, the incidence of discontinuation of ACEI therapy because of impairment in renal function has been low (1%–3%); in some studies, it was equivalent to that seen with placebo. The longer-acting ACEIs, however, may be associated with a higher risk of renal dysfunction.

Hyperkalemia An increase in serum potassium level can occur during ACEI therapy, and in some cases it may be significant enough to cause cardiac conduction abnormalities. The risk of hyperkalemia is significantly higher in patients with baseline renal dysfunction and/or when renal dysfunction occurs as a result of ACEI use. Continued use of potassium-sparing diuretics, potassium supplement, or salt substitute (that contains potassium) will obviously increase the risk of hyperkalemia. Concomitant use of aldosterone antagonists, especially in the presence of DM, is also associated with increased risk of hyperkalemia and can be reduced by appropriate dose adjustments.

Angioedema Angioedema is rare and occurs in less than 1% of patients taking ACEIs. It is well established that angioedema occurs far more frequently in blacks. Because angioedema may be life threatening, any history or clinical suspicion of such reactions in the past should be considered a contraindication for ACEI therapy. ARBs can be considered an alternative therapy because these agents are not thought to have a bradykinin-potentiating effect. However, such therapy should also be used with great caution in patients with ACEI-induced angioedema because there have been several reports of angioedema in patients who received ARB therapy.

ARBs

Several studies have shown that the RAS can have partial escape during long-term therapy with ACEIs, leading to increasing levels of angiotensin II despite continued therapy with ACEIs. This ACEI escape phenomenon occurs in part as a result of the alternative pathways for the production of angiotensin II that are localized in myocardial and vascular tissues (see **Fig. 3**). These alternate pathways (especially those that are chymase dependent) are activated in the setting of myocardial injury secondary to infarction.

Because ARBs provide direct blockade of angiotensin II type 1 receptors, they have been used to counteract angiotensin II produced by these alternate pathways. The use of ARBs results in the effective blockade of the potentially harmful effects of angiotensin II on tissues regardless of the site of origin of angiotensin II (see **Fig. 3**). In addition, this effect is achieved without accumulation of bradykinin, which is primarily responsible for some adverse reactions associated with the use of ACEIs, such as persistent cough, angioedema, and significant hypotension.

Theoretically, the use of these drugs should be associated with beneficial effects on clinical outcomes similar to those seen during ACEI therapy and with fewer side effects. The ARBs have produced favorable hemodynamic effects during short- and long-term administration. Also, randomized clinical trials comparing ARBs with ACEIs have generally shown equivalent or enhanced benefits.

Several ARBs have been evaluated in the setting of HF and are available for clinical use (see **Table 2**). Overall, several placebo-controlled studies have demonstrated that long-term therapy with ARBs is associated with beneficial effects on hemodynamic, neurohormonal, and clinical parameters that are expected with RAS blockade. However, the overall experience with ARBs in controlled clinical trials in HF is significantly less than that with ACEIs. Based on the clinical trial experience, at the present, only 3 ARBs are approved for the treatment of patients with HF (see **Table 2**). Although these ARBs can be considered an alternate RAS-blocking therapy, it is important to emphasize that ACEIs remain the first choice for inhibition of RAS in patients with HF. The use of ARBs should generally be reserved as an alternate therapy in patients who are intolerant to treatment with ACEIs. The benefit of alternative therapy with an ARB was well demonstrated (**Fig. 4**) with candesartan in the Candesartan in HF Assessment of Reduction in Mortality and Morbidity (CHARM) alternative trial.[10]

Practical considerations regarding the use of ARBs

Similar to the use of ACEIs, treatment with an ARB, when appropriate, should be started at low doses (see **Table 2**). In general, as discussed earlier, most of the considerations regarding the use of ARBs are similar to those with ACEIs. Close monitoring of blood pressure, renal function, and potassium level is recommended to start 1 to 2 weeks after the initiation of ARB therapy and as needed subsequently. Titration of ARB doses is generally achieved by doubling doses every 2 weeks until the target dose is achieved or the patient develops intolerance. The overall side effects related to the use of ARBs on renal function and serum potassium level are similar to those

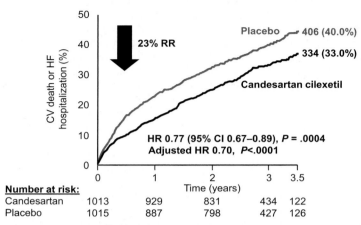

Fig. 4. Results of CHARM alternative study showing efficacy of candesartan versus placebo in patients with systolic heart failure. CHARM, Candesartan in Heart failure Assessment of Reduction in Mortality and Morbidity; CI, confidence interval; CV, cardiovascular; HR, hazard ratio; RR, relative risk. (*Adapted from* Granger CB, McMurray J, Yusuf S, et al. Effects of candesartan in patients with chronic heart failure and reduced left-ventricular systolic function intolerant to angiotensin-converting-enzyme inhibitors: the CHARM-Alternative trial. Lancet 2003;362:772–6.)

described earlier with ACEIs. However, angioedema (although reported in the literature) occurs rarely with ARBs.

Aldosterone receptor antagonists

With the activation of RAAS system as a result of cardiac dysfunction, there is significant increase in the levels of aldosterone, which leads to the activation of mineralocorticoid receptors and produces deleterious effects. Experimental data suggest that higher levels of aldosterone have a significant effect on cardiac structure and function that is independent and additive to the deleterious effects produced by angiotensin II. The deleterious effects associated with increased aldosterone levels include myocardial fibrosis secondary to increased collagen deposition, vascular inflammation and remodeling, salt and water retention, and loss of magnesium and potassium. Although treatment with ACEIs and ARBs initially lowers circulating levels of aldosterone for short periods of time, this effect is not sustained for a long period of time, leading to aldosterone escape. This has lead to the use of aldosterone blockade in the management of patients with HF who are already receiving treatment with ACEIs or ARBs and β-blockers.

In the Randomized ALdactone Evaluation Study (RALES), spironolactone was added to ACEI therapy for patients with New York Heart Association (NYHA) class III to IV HF who had been recently hospitalized. The treatment with spironolactone was associated with a 30% reduction the risk of death and a 35% reduction in HF hospitalization.[11] There was also a significant improvement in the overall functional status of patients treated with spironolactone. Based on these data, spironolactone is recommended as part of standard therapy for patients with NYHA class III or IV HF in addition to treatment with ACEIs/ARBs and β-blockers.

A subsequent study evaluated the newer and more specific aldosterone receptor antagonist eplerenone in patients with LVEF of 40% or less and clinical evidence of

HF or DM within 14 days of acute MI.[12] Treatment with eplerenone in addition to standard therapy including β-blockers and ACEIs/ARBs was associated with significant reduction in mortality and hospitalization for HF. Based on these findings, eplerenone is now recommended for post-MI patients with LV systolic dysfunction and HF or DM. A recent study in patients with LVEF of 35% or less and NYHA class II HF receiving standard therapy also demonstrated a significant benefit of treatment with eplerenone compared with placebo in reducing the risk of death and all-cause hospitalization and hospitalization for HF.[13]

Practical considerations Although the use of aldosterone antagonists can theoretically increase the risk of significant hyperkalemia (serum potassium >5.5 mEq/L) when properly used under close observation, the actual risk is low. However, because of the concern about hyperkalemia, it is generally recommended that the use of aldosterone receptor antagonists be carefully evaluated, taking into consideration the benefit versus risk, especially in patients with preexisting renal dysfunction, DM, and/or prior history of hyperkalemia. Special consideration needs to be given to the elderly, because serum creatinine might not be an accurate reflection of the renal function as a result of decreased muscle mass. Despite these limitations, it is strongly recommended that treatment with spironolactone should be considered in patients with NYHA class III or IV HF who are receiving adequate standard therapy with ACEIs/ARBs and β-blockers. The treatment should be generally started with the initial dosage of spironolactone 12.5 mg/d or eplerenone 25 mg/d, and renal function and potassium levels should be closely monitored. The development of potassium levels of greater than 5.5 mEq/L should lead to discontinuation and/or dose reduction of aldosterone receptor antagonists. Similarly, the development of worsening renal dysfunction should trigger careful evaluation and consideration for stopping aldosterone receptor antagonists. If no untoward side effects are encountered, the dosage should be gradually increased to the recommended target dose (see **Table 2**). Potassium supplementation should generally be stopped before the initiation of treatment except in rare instances when patients have required large amounts of potassium supplementation, in which case the dose of such supplements should be considerably lower. Salt substitutes also have a high potassium content and should be avoided. In addition, patients should be instructed to stop aldosterone receptor antagonists during an episode of gastroenteritis or while loop diuretic use is interrupted. Patients should also be cautioned to avoid the use of NSAIDs and cyclooxygenase 2 inhibitors because these agents increase the risk of hyperkalemia and renal dysfunction.

Inappropriate use of aldosterone receptor antagonists has been shown to be associated with significantly increased risk of hyperkalemia that may be associated with increased rates of hospitalization.

β-Blockers

Sympathetic adrenergic nervous system activation in response to cardiac dysfunction leads to higher levels of plasma catecholamines, which are associated with deleterious effects on the heart (see **Fig. 2**). Sympathetic activation causes profound vasoconstriction, leading to increased afterload, which subsequently increases ventricular pressures and volumes, thus perpetuating the process of cardiac remodeling. In addition, norepinephrine can itself induce cardiac hypertrophy and worsen myocardial ischemia in those with underlying CAD. Activation of SNS also impairs sodium excretion by the kidneys and promotes the release of aldosterone, which also leads to salt and water retention. Enhanced sympathetic activity can provoke arrhythmias by increasing the automaticity of myocytes, increasing trigger activity in the heart, and promoting electrolyte imbalance. High levels of norepinephrine also potentiate the actions of the RAAS. Finally, norepinephrine can trigger cardiac apoptosis by stimulating growth and increasing oxidative stress in terminally differentiated cells (see **Fig. 2**). It is because of these deleterious effects of the SNS activation in patients with HF that treatment with β-blockers was considered useful in HF despite their well-known negative inotropic effects. β-Blockers work primarily by preventing the adverse consequences of enhanced SNS activity in patients with HF, and these beneficial effects far outweigh their negative inotropic effects. Long-term studies with β-blockers have shown that continued use of β-blockers is associated with positive cardiac remodeling, which leads to significant improvement in LV performance associated with increased LVEF. There are several additional beneficial effects of β-blockers at the cellular level, which are beyond the scope of this review.

So far, only 3 β-blockers (carvedilol, bisoprolol, and sustained-release metoprolol succinate) have been shown to be effective (**Fig. 5**) in patients with chronic HF.[14–17] It is important to realize that the beneficial effects demonstrated with these 3 β-blockers do not indicate a β-blocker class effect, as shown by the lack of effectiveness of bucindolol and lack of effectiveness of short-acting metoprolol in clinical trials.[18,19]

β-Blockers have now been evaluated in numerous placebo-controlled clinical trials in patients with HF who have reduced LVEF (<35%–45%) and were already receiving treatment with diuretics and ACEIs, with or without digitalis. The aggregate experience from these trials indicates that long-term treatment with β-blockers reduced the symptoms of HF, improved the clinical status, and reduced the risk of hospitalization for HF. More important, in all trials, treatment with β-blocker was associated with a significant improvement in survival (see **Fig. 5**).[14–17] These benefits of β-blockers were seen in all subgroups of patients including those with milder or more severe HF, those with or without underlying CAD, those with or without DM, and black and female patients.

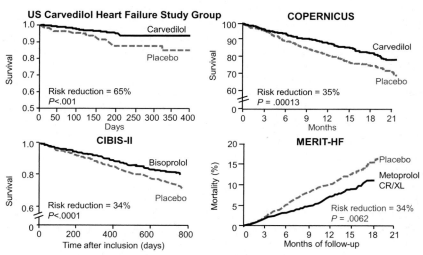

Fig. 5. Results of RCTs demonstrating effects of selected β-blocker therapy in patients with HF secondary to LV systolic dysfunction. CIBIS-II, Cardiac Insufficiency BIsoprolol Study II; COPERNICUS, CarvedilOl Prospective Randomized Cumulative Survival (COPERNICUS) study; MERIT-HF, MEtoprolol CR/XL Randomized Intervention Trial in congestive Heart Failure; RCT, randomized controlled trials. (*Adapted from* Refs.[14–17])

Practical considerations Based on the consistent efficacy and significant survival benefit of the 3 β-blockers approved for the treatment of HF, they are now recommended for all patients with chronic HF with reduced LVEF unless there is a contraindication or a history of intolerance. Because of the significant favorable effect of β-blockers on cardiac remodeling, disease progression, and survival, treatment with a β-blocker should be initiated as soon as evidence of LV dysfunction is demonstrated regardless of the severity of symptoms. This is true even when the patients have very mild symptoms and/or when, on subsequent treatment, they do not show improvement. The treatment with β-blocker should be continued and optimized to reduce the risk of progressive LV dysfunction and further clinical deterioration and prevent the risk of sudden cardiac death. The benefits of β-blocker therapy are evident even when the patient is not taking high doses of ACEIs. When both drugs cannot be used in maximal doses, the use of β-blocker has been shown to produce greater improvement in symptoms and reduction in risk of death in patients who are taking low-dose ACEI. Therefore, it seems prudent to optimize the dosage of β-blockers compared with maximizing the dosage of ACEIs, especially in patients who develop symptomatic hypotension with target doses of both classes of drugs.

Using β-blockers in the clinical setting β-Blocker therapy should generally be initiated in stable patients. Recent data show that β-blocker therapy can be started safely before discharge even in patients hospitalized with HF who did not require intravenous therapy for HF. It is not advisable to start β-blocker therapy in the presence of recently decompensated HF. Treatment with a β-blocker should be initiated at a very low dose (see **Table 2**). If a lower dose has been well tolerated, then the dose should be increased gradually, usually doubling the dose at 2-week intervals. Careful monitoring of heart rate, blood pressure, and HF symptoms is needed during the initial period and during the entire uptitration phase. All patients with current evidence or prior history of fluid retention should be on a diuretic before starting β-blocker therapy because diuretics are often needed to maintain sodium and fluid balance and prevent excessive fluid retention. Initiation of treatment with β-blocker can cause fluid retention and lead to decompensated HF. During this period, patients should be advised to weigh regularly on a daily basis and manage any weight increase by increasing the dose of diuretic to maintain the pretreatment weight. In the presence of significant fluid retention, planned increments in the dose of β-blocker should be delayed until the patient's clinical condition has been stabilized. With such a careful approach, most patients can tolerate the increase in dosing to the recommended target dose.

The optimal dose of β-blocker is the target dose achieved in the clinical trial. The target dose in the randomized controlled clinical trials was not based on the patients' therapeutic response but rather was dependent on a prespecified target dose. Lower doses were used in these trials only if the target dose could not be tolerated, and therefore most of these trials did not evaluate whether a lower dose would be effective. Thus, clinicians should make every effort to achieve the target dose of β-blocker shown to be effective in the clinical trials to ensure the maximal survival benefit in the given patient. Once the target dose has been reached, most patients can continue long-term therapy without difficulty. It is important to educate the patient that the clinical response to β-blocker therapy is generally delayed and may require many months of treatment before improvement is noted. Even when symptoms do not improve, long-term therapy with a β-blocker should be maintained to reduce the risk of major adverse clinical events. Abrupt withdrawal of β-blocker therapy is to be avoided because it can lead to clinical deterioration and β-blocker withdrawal syndrome. Because long-term treatment with a β-blocker reduces the risk of worsening HF, discontinuation of treatment with these drugs after an episode of decompensated HF will not diminish, and might increase, the subsequent risk of clinical decompensation. Therefore, even when patients develop fluid retention with or without worsening symptoms, it is advisable to continue β-blocker therapy and adjust the dose of diuretics. Only when the clinical deterioration is accompanied by hypoperfusion and/or requires the use of intravenous inotropic agents may it be necessary to decrease the dose or, in some cases, withhold β-blocker therapy temporarily until the patient's clinical status has been stabilized. Once stable, the β-blocker should be reintroduced to reduce the risk of worsening HF and adverse clinical outcome.

Safety and adverse experience As discussed earlier, initial therapy with β-blocker can cause fluid retention, which is generally asymptomatic but can occasionally lead to worsening of HF. Patients with fluid retention before treatment are at a higher risk of retaining fluid during the treatment, and thus the clinician should ensure that patients are euvolemic before initiating β-blocker therapy. As suggested earlier, any increase in weight or worsening signs and symptoms of HF should be quickly managed with an increased dosage of diuretic. However, the occurrence of fluid retention or decompensation of HF is generally not a reason for permanent withdrawal of β-blocker treatment.

Treatment with β-blocker can be associated with general fatigue and tiredness; therefore, it is important to educate the patients about such side effects in advance and ask them not to discontinue β-blocker therapy. Patient should be reassured that fatigue is generally short lasting and resolves within a few weeks of initiation of β-blocker therapy. In some cases, the fatigue may be significant enough to limit further increment in dose and, rarely, may require a reduction if symptoms are severe. But treatment should not be discontinued unless there is evidence of hypoperfusion.

Bradycardia and slowing of cardiac conduction are expected effects of β-blockers. In most patients, bradycardia is asymptomatic and requires no treatments. However, if high-grade (second- or third-degree) atrioventicular block develops, the dose of β-blocker should be reduced and careful evaluation should be made regarding other conditions or agents that can cause bradycardia or heart block. In some cases when bradycardia persists and is significant, consideration of pacemaker therapy to permit the use of β-blocker may be reasonable.

Although hypotension can occur with β-blocker therapy (especially with carvedilol because of its α-blocking action), it is usually asymptomatic. When hypotension is associated with dizziness, lightheadedness, or blurred vision, it might be necessary to reduce the dose and/or change the β-blocker to a non–α-blocking agent. The risk of hypotension can also be minimized by administering β-blockers and ACEIs/ARBs at different times of the day. If hypotension persists, a decrease in the dose of ACEI/ARB might be necessary, and in some cases the dose of diuretic might need to be reduced in patients who are volume depleted.

Vasodilator therapy

Although vasodilator therapy was beneficial and extensively used several decades ago, since the introduction of ACEIs in conjunction with diuretic therapy, treatment with oral vasodilators is not considered necessary in most patients with chronic HF. However, there are special situations where recent data demonstrate that combined vasodilator therapy with hydralazine–isosorbide dinitrate can provide significant additional benefit to that achieved during standard therapy with ACEIs and β-blockers. In the African-American Heart Failure Trial (A-HeFT), which enrolled self-described African American patients with HF who remained symptomatic despite optimal

Table 3
Relative benefits of various evidence-based drug therapies for HF

Guideline-Suggested Therapy	RRR,% (RCT)	RRR,% (meta-analyses)
ACEI/ARB	17	20%
β-Blocker	34	31%
Aldosterone antagonist	30	25%
Hydralazine–nitrate	43	NA

Abbreviations: NA, not applicable; RCT, randomized clinical trials; RRR, relative risk reduction.
Adapted from Fonarow G, Yancy C, Hernandez A, et al. Potential impact of optimal implementation of evidence-based heart failure therapies on mortality. Am Heart J 2011;161:1024.

medical therapy, treatment with the combination of hydralazine and isosorbide dinitrate was associated with significant improvement in survival (43% decrease in mortality rate).[20] This benefit was presumed to be related to enhanced nitric oxide bioavailability (which is thought to be decreased in African American patients). Based on these data, the guidelines now recommend treatment with fixed combination of hydralazine and isosorbide dinitrate (see **Table 2**) in African American patients who remain symptomatic despite optimal standard therapy for HF. Although there is paucity of data with this vasodilator combination in other individuals with HF, it might be considered as a therapeutic option in patients who are intolerant of ACEIs.

Clinical application of evidence-based therapy
Despite the overwhelming evidence of benefits with evidence-based therapy using RAAS-blocking drugs and β-blocking agents in patients with HF and LV systolic dysfunction, their application in clinical practice is less than ideal. The burden of HF is enormous and increasing in the United States. HF remains a leading cause of hospitalization in the United States. In addition, the patients with HF suffer from significant morbidity and mortality. All of these consequences of HF can be substantially reduced by adequate implementation of evidence-based therapy that is recommended by all guidelines. A recent analysis emphasized the degree of benefit in reducing mortality that can be achieved with the use of evidence-based therapy in patients with HF **(Table 3)**.[21] This analysis also emphasized that optimal implementation of evidence-based therapies with ACEIs/ARBs, β-blockers, aldosterone antagonists, and hydralazine–isosorbide dinitrate combination could potentially prevent as many as 47,500 deaths per year in the United States. These data clearly emphasize that considerable opportunity exists for the implementation of evidence-based therapy in patient with HF caused by LV systolic dysfunction to improve the associated adverse prognosis.

REFERENCES

1. Hunt SA, Abraham WT, Chin MH, et al. 2009 Focused update incorporated into the ACC/AHA 2005 guidelines for the diagnosis and management of heart failure in adults: a report of the American College of Cardiology Foundation/American Heart Association Task Force on Practice Guidelines. Circulation 2009;119: e391–479.
2. Lindenfeld J, Albert NM, Boehmer JP, et al. HFSA 2010 comprehensive heart failure practice guideline. J Card Fail 2010;16:e1–194.
3. CONSENSUS Trial Study Group: effects of enalapril on mortality in severe congestive heart failure: results of the Cooperative North Scandinavian Enalapril Survival Study (CONSENSUS). N Engl J Med 1987;316:1429–35.

4. SOLVD investigators: effect on enalapril on survival in patients with reduced left ventricular ejection fractions and congestive heart failure. N Engl J Med 1991; 325:293–302.

5. SOLVD Investigators. Effect of enalapril on mortality and the development of heart failure in asymptomatic patients with reduced left ventricular ejection fractions. N Engl J Med 1992;327:685–91.

6. Pfeffer M, Braunwald E, Moye L, et al. Effect of captopril on mortality and morbidity in patients with left ventricular dysfunction after myocardial infarction. Results of the survival and ventricular enlargement trial. The SAVE Investigators. N Engl J Med 1992;327:669–77.

7. Acute Infarction Ramipril Efficacy (AIRE) Study Investigators. Effect of ramipril on mortality and morbidity of survivors of acute myocardial infarction with clinical evidence of heart failure. Lancet 1993;342:821–8.

8. Køber L, Torp-Pedersen C, Carlsen JE, et al. A clinical trial of the angiotensin-converting-enzyme inhibitor trandolapril in patients with left ventricular dysfunction after myocardial infarction. Trandolapril Cardiac Evaluation (TRACE) Study Group. N Engl J Med 1995;333(25):1670–6.

9. Ambrosioni E, Borghi C, Magnani B. The effect of the angiotensin-converting-enzyme inhibitor zofenopril on mortality and morbidity after anterior myocardial infarction. The Survival of Myocardial Infarction Long-Term Evaluation (SMILE) Study Investigators. N Engl J Med 1995;332(2):80–5.

10. Granger C, McMurray J, Yusuf S, et al, CHARM Investigators and Committees. Effects of candesartan in patients with chronic heart failure and reduced left-ventricular systolic function intolerant to angiotensin-converting-enzyme inhibitors: the CHARM-Alternative trial. Lancet 2003;362:772–6.

11. Pitt B, Zannad F, Remme WJ, et al. The effect of spironolactone on morbidity and mortality in patients with severe heart failure. Randomized Aldactone Evaluation Study Investigators. N Engl J Med 1999;341(10):709–17.

12. Pitt B, Remme W, Zannad F, et al, Eplerenone Post-Acute Myocardial Infarction Heart Failure Efficacy and Survival Study Investigators. Eplerenone, a selective aldosterone blocker, in patients with left ventricular dysfunction after myocardial infarction. N Engl J Med 2003;348(14):1309–21.

13. Zannad F, McMurray J, Krum H, et al, EMPHASIS-HF Study Group. Eplerenone in patients with systolic heart failure and mild symptoms. N Engl J Med 2011;364: 11–21.

14. Packer M, Bristow MR, Cohn JN, et al. The effect of carvedilol on morbidity and mortality in patients with chronic heart failure. U.S. Carvedilol Heart Failure Study Group. N Engl J Med 1996;334:1349–55.

15. Packer M, Coats AJ, Fowler MB, et al, Carvedilol Prospective Randomized Cumulative Survival Study Group (COPERNICUS). Effect of carvedilol on survival in severe chronic heart failure. N Engl J Med 2001;344:1651–8.

16. CIBIS-II investigators and committees: the Cardiac Insufficiency Bisoprolol Study II (CIBIS-II): A randomized trial. Lancet 1999;353:9–13.

17. Effect of metoprolol CR/XL in chronic heart failure: metoprolol CR/XL Randomised Intervention Trial in Congestive Heart Failure (MERIT-HF). Lancet 1999;353: 2001–7.

18. Beta-Blocker Evaluation of Survival Trial Investigators. A trial of the beta-blocker bucindolol in patients with advanced chronic heart failure. N Engl J Med 2001; 344:1659–67.

19. Poole-Wilson P, Swedberg K, Cleland J, et al, COMET investigators. Comparison of carvedilol and metoprolol on clinical outcomes in patients with chronic heart

failure in the Carvedilol Or Metoprolol European Trial (COMET): randomised controlled trial. Lancet 2003;362:7–13.

20. Taylor AL, Ziesche S, Yancy C, et al, African-American Heart Failure Trial Investigators. Combination of isosorbide dinitrate and hydralazine in blacks with heart failure. N Engl J Med 2004;351(20):2049–57.

21. Fonarow G, Yancy C, Hernandez A, et al. Potential impact of optimal implementation of evidence-based heart failure therapies on mortality. Am Heart J 2011; 161:1024–1030.e3.

Diuretics in Heart Failure
Practical Considerations

Jagroop Basraon, DO[a], Prakash C. Deedwani, MD[a,b],*

KEYWORDS

• Diuretics • Heart failure • Loop diuretics • Diuretic resistance

KEY POINTS

• Diuretics are essential medications for volume control in patients with acute and chronic heart failure.
• Diuretic use can lead to significant electrolyte disturbances, including hypokalemia. This needs to be monitored and corrected to prevent arrhythmogenic complications.
• Combination therapy can be used to enhance the effectiveness of diuretic therapy.
• Cardiorenal syndrome may develop in patients on chronic diuretic therapy. This can be attenuated with use of Renin-Angiotensin-Aldosterone System blocking drugs.

INTRODUCTION

Treatment with diuretic therapy is an essential component in the treatment of a wide spectrum of heart failure presentations. It is commonly used as the first-line therapy for the treatment of acute decompensation as well as chronic treatment of heart failure to help maintain a euvolemic state. Practitioners in every specialty of medicine are exposed to patients with chronic heart failure for the management of comorbid conditions; therefore, an in-depth understanding of diuretic therapy is essential in optimizing patient care.

This review discusses the role of diuretics in heart failure by focusing on different classifications and mechanisms of action. Pharmacodynamic and pharmacokinetic properties of diuretics are elucidated. The predominant discussion highlights the use of loop diuretics, which are the most commonly used drugs in heart failure. Different methods of using this therapy in different settings along with a comprehensive review of the side-effect profile are highlighted. Special situations necessitating adjustment and the phenomenon of diuretic resistance are explained.

MECHANISM OF ACTION

Diuretics with different modes of action are available for heart failure therapy. They are classified based on different sites of action within the nephron. A pharmacologic

[a] University of California-San Francisco, Fresno, CA, USA; [b] Cardiology Division, Veterns Affairs Central California Health Care System, E224, 2615 E Clinton Avenue, Fresno, CA 93703, USA
* Corresponding author.
E-mail address: deed@fresno.ucsf.edu

Med Clin N Am 96 (2012) 933–942
http://dx.doi.org/10.1016/j.mcna.2012.07.003
0025-7125/12/$ – see front matter © 2012 Published by Elsevier Inc.

medical.theclinics.com

effect is achieved because of their inhibition of electrolyte transporters, which causes a corresponding hemodynamic effect because of the alteration of the interstitial tonicity and loss of fluid caused by osmotic gradients (**Fig. 1**). Diuretics are tightly bound to plasma proteins and, therefore, restricted to the intravascular space. They are actively secreted into the proximal tubular lumen. Loop diuretics inhibit the Na+/K+/Cl- symporter in the ascending loop of Henle, whereas thiazide-type diuretics affect the Na+/Cl- in the distal convoluted tubules. Potassium-sparing diuretics and mineralocorticoid receptor antagonists, which are used more for concomitant therapeutics as renin-angiotensin-aldosterone system (RAAS) blocking agents and in the reduction of diuretic-induced hypokalemia instead of the control of edema, work at sites in the collecting duct to inhibit the Na+/K+ transporter.

PHARMACOKINETICS

Loop diuretics have different pharmacokinetic properties depending on the diuretic used and patients' underlying comorbidities (**Table 1**). Particularly, patients with kidney and liver disease can be challenging to manage because of varied elimination and altered metabolisms.

Orally dosed furosemide typically has 50% bioavailability; however, significant variability has been reported, with a range from 10% to 100% in patients with heart failure.[1] Bumetanide and torsemide, the newer agents are absorbed more completely with 80% bioavailability after oral dosing.[2,3] Hydrochlorothiazide- and thiazide-type diuretic metolazone have reported bioavailability of 60% to 70%.[4] Furosemide is eliminated by the kidneys, whereas torsemide and bumetanide are metabolized by the liver. Metolazone and thiazides are all eliminated by renal mechanisms.[4] Loop diuretics typically have short half-lives, with Bumex at about 3 to 4 hours, 1 to 2 hours for torsemide, and 2 to 3 hours for furosemide. Thiazides typically stay in the system longer, with an average half-life of 10 to 15 hours.[5]

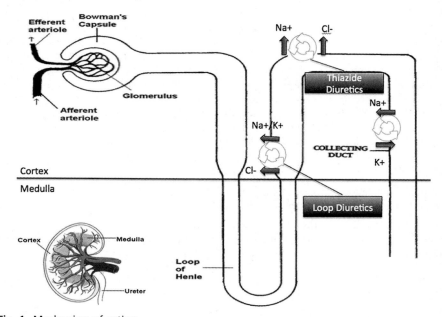

Fig. 1. Mechanism of action.

Table 1
Pharmacology of diuretics

	Oral Bioavailability (%)	Dosing (mg)	Half-Life (Hours)	Elimination
LOOP				
Furosemide	0–100	80–160	2	Renal
Torsemide	80–100	10–20	1	Liver
Bumetanide	80–100	2–4	3	Liver
Other				
Hydrochlorothiazide	65–75	12.5–100.0	6–15	Renal
Metolazone	70–85	2.5–10.0	14	Renal

DIURETICS IN RENAL AND LIVER DISEASE

These characteristics have an important impact in the management of patients with hepatic or renal disease. Presence of renal dysfunction caused by underlying kidney disease or secondary to hypoperfusion because of chronic heart failure can lead to altered pharmacokinetics, which requires adjustment of the diuretic dose to ensure an adequate dose response.

In patients with renal disease, there is decreased renal flow and often decreased production of urine in the later stages. Physiologic alterations also lead to decreased renal conjugation. Regardless of the specific kidney disease, the functioning nephrons remain responsive to diuretic therapy. These changes necessitate the use of higher doses of the loop diuretic to achieve adequate concentration in the tubular fluid to be effective. Additionally, this results in the increased half-life of furosemide, which is renally excreted; however, bumetanide and torsemide are not affected due to their hepatic metabolism.[6]

The predominant diuretic used in patients with liver disease without heart failure is spironolactone. This diuretic is predominantly used because the volume problems are manifestations of hyperaldosteronism.[7] The response of loop diuretics is reduced in patients with liver disease with heart failure.[8] Typically, spironolactone is used with additional low-dose hydrochlorothiazide or intra-abdominal procedures, such as paracentesis, to control fluid status. These patients can often suffer from intravascular fluid depletion, therefore, the addition of a loop diuretic has to be carefully used. In these patients, the amount of fluid excretion is lower because of the shift of the natriuretic curve to the right and cannot be overcome with larger doses. Lastly, the frequency of the response is not affected; thus, multiple doses may be used to increase urine output.[9] Therefore, frequent dosing or combination therapy can overcome some of this decrease.

PHARMACODYNAMICS

Pharmacodynamics of diuretics can be evaluated by an indirect measurement of the rate of excretion within the urine. Typically, this relationship is represented by a sigmoidal curve whereby a minimal amount of diuretic is required to achieve a renal response with an upper level for maximal effect (**Fig. 2**).[3,10] These dose response curves have helped established the optimal dose limits of the commonly used diuretics[2,11–13] Therefore, it is important to keep in mind that the clinical application of the diuretic usually requires a minimal dose before an effective diuresis can be established.

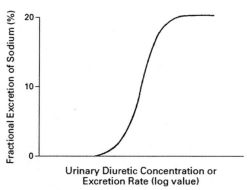

Fig. 2. Pharmacodynamics of loop diuretics. The relation between the natriuretic response and the amount of diuretic reaching the site of action is represented by a sigmoid curve. (*Modified from* Brater DC. Diuretic therapy. N Engl J Med 1998;339(6):387–95.)

DOSING

Diuretics are typically administered on a schedule, which accounts for their different half-lives. Loop diuretics are dosed twice a day because of typical (1–4 hours) half-lives. Thiazides and metolazone typically have the longest half-lives and, therefore, are dosed daily. Patients presenting with evidence of volume overload are typically started on 40 mg of furosemide twice a day and observed for a diuretic response. In case of inadequate diuresis or those on chronic therapy, the patients' basal dose is adjusted to increase urine output.

INTRAVENOUS THERAPY

Intravenous loop diuretics are the most commonly used medication during acute decompensated heart failure. Intravenous dosing forms of certain diuretics are available for therapy and are usually equivalent in efficacy to the oral form, with the exception of furosemide whereby half of the oral dose should be used in the intravenous format because of bioavailability differences.

BOLUS VERSUS CONTINUOUS DOSING

There has been a contentious debate over the effectiveness of different methods of administering intravenous diuretics. Additionally, there have been concerns over the adverse effects of using high doses of diuretics in patients' with heart failure.[14] The comparison of bolus versus continuous dosing in several older studies did not clearly establish superiority of either method.[15–17] However, recently a randomized clinical trial has provided further information in this regard.

In the DOSE (Diuretic Strategies in patients with Acute Decompensated Heart Failure) trial, which was a prospective randomized controlled trial, different strategies of applying diuretic therapy in patients with clinical heart failure were evaluated.[18] Patients were evaluated at a low dose versus a high dose, which was defined as 2.5 times their usual daily therapeutic dose both in an intravenous and continuous infusion methods during acute decompensated heart failure. There was no difference in the kidney function and in the overall assessment of heart failure symptoms between the two treatment strategies (**Fig. 3**). Therefore, based on results of this study either mode of administration can be used with appropriate clinical monitoring.

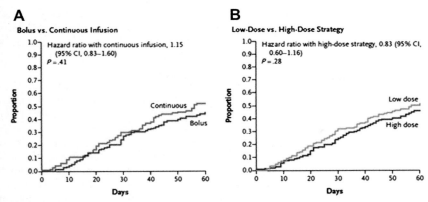

Fig. 3. Kaplan-Meier curves for the clinical composite end point of death, rehospitalization, or emergency department visit. CI, confidence interval. (*Modified from* Felker GM, Lee KL, Bull DA, et al. Diuretic strategies in patients with acute decompensated heart failure. N Engl J Med 2011;364(9):797–805.)

COMBINATION THERAPY

In patients with high-dose diuretic requirements or a worsening response caused by diuretic resistance, combination therapy can be used to increase diuretic efficacy. Commonly, metolazone or HCTZ is added as a single dose to the scheduled loop diuretic dosing.[19] This combination has proved to be efficacious in multiple conditions, including heart failure and liver disease, independent of age.[20,21] This strategy uses a sequential blockade of the electrolyte transporters, which counteracts the chronic adaptions of the nephrons to the previously prescribed diuretic therapy. Although this strategy has never been tested in large randomized clinical trials, smaller studies of up to 300 patients have demonstrated positive outcomes.[22]

Optimal candidates for combination therapy include those with advanced kidney disease, high oral dose requirements of loop diuretics, advanced heart failure with multiple repeated hospitalizations, as well as those with acute decompensation refractory to intravenous diuretics. Such combination therapy also requires the consideration of patients' electrolyte status as arrhythmogenic complications from hypokalemia can occur and are preventable with adequate supplementation or the use of potassium-sparing diuretic therapy.[23]

DIURETIC RESISTANCE

Diuretic use is associated with 2 important physiologic phenomena that are important to understand when using diuretics for chronic therapy. These phenomena include the diuretic braking phenomenon and the development of diuretic resistance with longer duration of therapy. These mechanisms are not independent but likely a combination or interrelated adaptation in response to the diuretic therapy.[24]

After the initial diuretic treatment, the repeated dose of the diuretic results in the retention of sodium to compensate for the volume contraction. This retention results in decreasing natruresis following each administration, with an eventual return to the preadministration levels. Additionally, over the long term, many adaptations in the tubular microchannels result in the decreasing efficacy of the diuretic, with requirements for higher dosing and the need for continuous or concurrent administration of another diuretic to maintain an effective response.[25] Therefore, patients on stable doses who begin to require titration of their current therapy may be candidates for the previously mentioned combination therapy or alternative approaches for the maintenance of the euvolemic state.

ADVERSE EFFECTS

Diuretics are effective agents for volume control in patients with heart failure. However, this potent effect comes at the cost of several common side effects. In addition to the expected volume depletion, several electrolyte abnormalities are commonly identified. These include difficulty with the maintenance of adequate serum potassium concentration. Hyponatremia, which is often multifactorial in patients with heart failure, can be exacerbated. Additionally, magnesium and calcium irregularities can also occur. Uric acid levels leading to hyperuricemia, which can exacerbate underlying crystalloid arthritides (Gout), has also be identified as a potential complication. Lastly, dose-related ototoxicity is a well-known complication that requires careful monitoring because of the potential for permanent damage.

As expected, any agent that results in the net loss of fluid will result in the reduction of intravascular volume with associated clinical findings. Overdiuresis can frequently lead to states of hypoperfusion, especially in the elderly or patients who are dependent or debilitated. Clinical sequelae from the organ affected by hypoperfusion can lead to some very common presentations. These include acute renal failure and hypotension with altered mentation, which is often compounded if patients are on concurrent anti-hypertensive therapy. Additionally, factors, such as limited fluid intake, fluid loss from diarrhea, or other systemic illness, can further compromise the normal intravascular volume. Also, initiation and/or uptitration of RAAS (renin-angiotension-aldosterone-system) blocking drugs can be associated with hypotension specially inn certain patients who has overactive RAAS phenomenon secondary to diuresis. This scenario can be easily remedied with the use of gentle fluid hydration with isotonic saline or increased oral intake.

Hypokalemia is one of the most frequent complications of diuretic therapy.[26] Physiologic design of the nephron and the effect of aldosterone are responsible for this finding. Decreased absorption of the sodium establishes an increased sodium gradient in the nephron, which leads to increased potassium secretion when this sodium load reaches the distal part of the nephron. Additionally, volume depletion leads to increased secretion of aldosterone in an attempt to retain sodium and that leads to further potassium loss.[27] The loss of the chloride ion has also been implicated as a potential reason for hypokalemia. Higher doses of diuretics are generally associated with lower potassium levels. However, a direct dose response cannot be clearly established because of the variability in diet and the effect of other concurrent factors, such as medication and other active disease processes.

The threshold of treatment of hypokalemia in patients with diuretic therapy is often determined by a number of factors. These factors include serum potassium concentration, whereby potassium levels less than 3.5 mmol/L indicates significantly decreased potassium stores. Additionally, cardiac arrhythmogenic complications caused by hypokalemia (specially in patients on digital glycosides) often require acute and chronic treatment to maintain adequate levels. Another option, depending on a compelling indication, is the addition of a potassium-sparing diuretic or aldosterone-blocking agent, which can counteract the expected potassium loss. Regardless of the strategy, close clinical monitoring of patients is required to achieve the desired diuresis and to minimize electrolyte complications.

Uric acid levels can be adversely affected by the use of diuretic therapy.[28] Although most patients with diuretic-induced hyperuricemia are asymptomatic, an attack of gout can be precipitated on the initiation of diuretic therapy.[29] Diuretic therapy can often be continued with acute treatment of the gout episode and monitoring of uric acid level trends.

Hyponatremia in patients treated with heart failure is associated with adverse outcomes.[30] No single factor can be identified and it is likely a result of multiple systems acting on the kidney that interfere with fluid excretion. Diuretics can exacerbate hyponatremia because alterations in the concentration gradient can impair the urinary-diluting ability.

Ototoxicity is another serious complication of high-dose loop diuretic therapy and the failure to recognize it can lead to permanent sensory damage. It is presumed that toxicity is mediated by an alteration in the electrochemical gradients in the lymphatics of the inner ear. Toxicity is directly related to the level and rate of accumulation of the diuretic in the serum. Rapid bolus injection or large amounts of daily dosing increases the likelihood of ototoxicity. Empiric data indicates that this damage is most often reversible if it is recognized in a timely fashion and the diuretic held or reduced. Additionally, it is much more common with older diuretic ethacrynic acid instead of furosemide or bumetanide.

CARDIORENAL SYNDROME

Adverse effects on kidney function in patients with heart failure have led to an emerging concept of cardiorenal syndrome. It is considered to be a complex process that is likely multifactorial in cause.[31] Several of these factors can be attributed to concurrent diuretic use. Experimental studies have indicated that the use of diuretics is associated with increased stimulation of the renal-angiotensin syndrome with increased levels of aldosterone. Animal studies have demonstrated that these changes can lead to increased renal fibrosis.[32] Additionally, other physiologic factors, such as anemia, increased sympathetic tone, oxidative stress, and endothelial dysfunction, are under investigation as potential therapeutic targets for reduction in cardiorenal syndrome because they are associated with detrimental vascular changes within the kidneys in patients with heart failure.[33,34] Therefore, a neurohormonal consequences of diuretics needs to be understood, and appropriate therapy with RAAS blocking agents needs to be implemented concurrently with diuretic use to mitigate the chronic and often irreversible deterioration of the renal system, which is essential in maintaining volume control in patients with heart failure.

GUIDELINES

Clear recommendations for diuretic therapy have been issued in the guidelines from the Heart Failure Society of American regarding use in acute and chronic heart failure. In chronic care, loop diuretics are recommended as class I agents to control fluid and relieve congestion, with level of evidence A for oral and intravenous therapy. Thiazide-type diuretics are described as second-line agents with class I and level of evidence B. Combination therapy carries a class II and level of evidence C. In cases of acute decompensation, the society recommends intravenous therapy with loop diuretic as class I with level of evidence B.

NEWER AGENTS

Recently, a vasopressin antagonist tolvaptan has been approved for use in patients with hyponatremia. Hyponatremia is often caused by chronic fluid retention in patients with heart failure and associated with adverse outcomes.[35] This agent counteracts the antidiuretic properties of the human hormone vasopressin which is increased in patients with heart failure.[36] The initial trials did include patients with hyponatremia from heart failure but they were not designed to address the net clinical benefit in this population as discussed by Cole and colleagues elsewhere in this issue.

Currently, the role of this medication continues to evolve and may assume greater importance with further studies in patients with heart failure.

SUMMARY

Diuretic therapy is an essential component for the control of heart failure symptoms and to prevent the morbidity and mortality associated with this condition. They are effective agents that cause diuresis by altering the osmotic gradients in the kidney and help generate net fluid loss. Liver and kidney disease can affect the pharmacologic properties, and patients' profiles need to be evaluated before their application.

Different routes of administration are available depending on the clinical presentation, and no particular type of administration has been shown to be superior to others in patients with heart failure. Prolonged use can result in resistance and requires application in combinations and the titration of dosing to get the desired effect.

These agents are not risk free and close patient monitoring is necessary for successful application. Hypokalemia is the most frequent electrolyte abnormality, which can be associated with significant mortality (due to risk of arrhythmia) if not properly recognized. Over time, the effectiveness of diuretic therapy is diminished because of the adverse remodeling of the renal system from hormonal disturbances caused by heart failure. This entity, known as the cardiorenal system, can make it difficult to control patients' volume status with diuretics. However, proper use of diuretic therapy with concurrently aggressive heart failure treatment (RAAS blockade) can ensure the effectiveness of diuretics.

The clinical practice guidelines have also recognized the use of diuretics of different combinations and in different scenarios and have given strong and specific recommendations to advance the evidence-based care of patients with heart failure. Lastly, newer agents are under investigation with the recent approval of a vasopressin antagonist to reduce hyponatremia from chronic fluid overload states in heart failure.

In summary, diuretics were the first agents to be used in the care of patients with heart failure. Proper understanding of their role and applying them in an evidence-based manner will help reduce the burden of heart failure for our society.

REFERENCES

1. Vargo DL, Kramer WG, Black PK, et al. Bioavailability, pharmacokinetics, and pharmacodynamics of torsemide and furosemide in patients with congestive heart failure. Clin Pharmacol Ther 1995;57(6):601–9.
2. Brater DC, Leinfelder J, Anderson SA. Clinical pharmacology of torsemide, a new loop diuretic. Clin Pharmacol Ther 1987;42(2):187–92.
3. Brater DC, Chennavasin P, Day B, et al. Bumetanide and furosemide. Clin Pharmacol Ther 1983;34(2):207–13.
4. Welling PG. Pharmacokinetics of the thiazide diuretics. Biopharm Drug Dispos 1986;7(6):501–35.
5. Beermann B, Groschinsky-Grind M, Rosen A. Absorption, metabolism, and excretion of hydrochlorothiazide. Clin Pharmacol Ther 1976;19(5 Pt 1):531–7.
6. Huang CM, Atkinson AJ Jr, Levin M, et al. Pharmacokinetics of furosemide in advanced renal failure. Clin Pharmacol Ther 1974;16(4):659–66.
7. Hou W, Sanyal AJ. Ascites: diagnosis and management. Med Clin North Am 2009;93(4):801–17, vii.

8. Fuller R, Hoppel C, Ingalls ST. Furosemide kinetics in patients with hepatic cirrhosis with ascites. Clin Pharmacol Ther 1981;30(4):461–7.

9. Villeneuve JP, Verbeeck RK, Wilkinson GR, et al. Furosemide kinetics and dynamics in patients with cirrhosis. Clin Pharmacol Ther 1986;40(1):14–20.

10. Chennavasin P, Seiwell R, Brater DC. Pharmacokinetic-dynamic analysis of the indomethacin-furosemide interaction in man. J Pharmacol Exp Ther 1980; 215(1):77–81.

11. Chennavasin P, Seiwell R, Brater DC, et al. Pharmacodynamic analysis of the furosemide-probenecid interaction in man. Kidney Int 1979;16(2):187–95.

12. Cook JA, Smith DE, Cornish LA, et al. Kinetics, dynamics, and bioavailability of bumetanide in healthy subjects and patients with congestive heart failure. Clin Pharmacol Ther 1988;44(5):487–500.

13. Brater DC. Diuretic therapy. N Engl J Med 1998;339(6):387–95.

14. Mielniczuk LM, Tsang SW, Desai AS, et al. The association between high-dose diuretics and clinical stability in ambulatory chronic heart failure patients. J Card Fail 2008;14(5):388–93.

15. Thomson MR, Nappi JM, Dunn SP, et al. Continuous versus intermittent infusion of furosemide in acute decompensated heart failure. J Card Fail 2010;16(3):188–93.

16. Dormans TP, van Meyel JJ, Gerlag PG, et al. Diuretic efficacy of high dose furosemide in severe heart failure: bolus injection versus continuous infusion. J Am Coll Cardiol 1996;28(2):376–82.

17. Allen LA, Turer AT, Dewald T, et al. Continuous versus bolus dosing of furosemide for patients hospitalized for heart failure. Am J Cardiol 2010;105(12):1794–7.

18. Felker GM, Lee KL, Bull DA, et al. Diuretic strategies in patients with acute decompensated heart failure. N Engl J Med 2011;364(9):797–805.

19. Sica DA. Metolazone and its role in edema management. Congest Heart Fail 2003;9(2):100–5.

20. Ghose RR, Gupta SK. Synergistic action of metolazone with "loop" diuretics. Br Med J (Clin Res Ed) 1981;282(6274):1432–3.

21. Brater DC, Pressley RH, Anderson SA. Mechanisms of the synergistic combination of metolazone and bumetanide. J Pharmacol Exp Ther 1985;233(1): 70–4.

22. Jentzer JC, DeWald TA, Hernandez AF. Combination of loop diuretics with thiazide-type diuretics in heart failure. J Am Coll Cardiol 2010;56(19):1527–34.

23. Cooper HA, Dries DL, Davis CE, et al. Diuretics and risk of arrhythmic death in patients with left ventricular dysfunction. Circulation 1999;100(12):1311–5.

24. Stanton BA, Kaissling B. Adaptation of distal tubule and collecting duct to increased Na delivery. II. Na+ and K+ transport. Am J Physiol 1988;255(6 Pt 2): F1269–75.

25. Kobayashi S, Clemmons DR, Nogami H, et al. Tubular hypertrophy due to work load induced by furosemide is associated with increases of IGF-1 and IGFBP-1. Kidney Int 1995;47(3):818–28.

26. Greenberg A. Diuretic complications. Am J Med Sci 2000;319(1):10–24.

27. Tannen RL. Diuretic-induced hypokalemia. Kidney Int 1985;28(6):988–1000.

28. Helgeland A, Hjermann I, Holme I, et al. Serum triglycerides and serum uric acid in untreated and thiazide-treated patients with mild hypertension. The Oslo study. Am J Med 1978;64(1):34–8.

29. Johnson MW, Mitch WE. The risks of asymptomatic hyperuricaemia and the use of uricosuric diuretics. Drugs 1981;21(3):220–5.

30. Klein L, O'Connor CM, Leimberger JD, et al. Lower serum sodium is associated with increased short-term mortality in hospitalized patients with worsening heart

failure: results from the Outcomes of a Prospective Trial of Intravenous Milrinone for Exacerbations of Chronic Heart Failure (OPTIME-CHF) study. Circulation 2005;111(19):2454–60.

31. Bock JS, Gottlieb SS. Cardiorenal syndrome: new perspectives. Circulation 2010; 121(23):2592–600.
32. Brilla CG, Pick R, Tan LB, et al. Remodeling of the rat right and left ventricles in experimental hypertension. Circulation 1990;67(6):1355–64.
33. Vesey DA, Cheung C, Pat B, et al. Erythropoietin protects against ischaemic acute renal injury. Nephrol Dial Transplant 2004;19(2):348–55.
34. Tojo A, Onozato ML, Kobayashi N, et al. Angiotensin II and oxidative stress in Dahl salt-sensitive rat with heart failure. Hypertension 2002;40(6):834–9.
35. Gheorghiade M, Abraham WT, Albert NM, et al. Relationship between admission serum sodium concentration and clinical outcomes in patients hospitalized for heart failure: an analysis from the OPTIMIZE-HF registry. Eur Heart J 2007;28(8):980–8.
36. Schrier RW, Gross P, Gheorghiade M, et al. Tolvaptan, a selective oral vaso-pressin V2-receptor antagonist, for hyponatremia. N Engl J Med 2006;355(20): 2099–112.

Inotropic Therapy
An Important Role in the Treatment of Advanced Symptomatic Heart Failure

Patrick McCann, MD, Paul J. Hauptman, MD*

KEYWORDS

- Inotropic therapy • Heart failure • Low cardiac output syndrome

KEY POINTS

- Inotropic therapy remains an option in the management of patients with advanced heart failure symptoms due to systolic dysfunction who do not respond to conventional therapies.
- The decision to use this class is largely predicated on an accurate evaluation of the patient's fluid and perfusion status.
- Selection of the appropriate agent and dosing regimens requires an understanding of the underlying pathophysiology of heart failure and concomitant therapy. Most important, the goals of care should be stated clearly, given inherent risks associated with this class of drug.

Acute decompensated heart failure is a highly prevalent condition, accounting for more than 1 million admissions in the United States per year.[1] However, it is a difficult clinical syndrome to precisely define. The current working definition of heart failure as promulgated by the Heart Failure Society of America is comprehensive (**Box 1**) but lacks specificity. Acute or acute-on-chronic presentations require a focused history and physical examination aimed at assessing volume status, peripheral perfusion, exacerbating factors, comorbidities, and prognosis; synthesizing these complex data points can lead to an appropriate selection of care options. This article provides an overview of the approach to the patient and focuses on the need for and timing of intravenous inotropic therapy, an important yet infrequently selected treatment generally reserved for patients for whom more conventional approaches fail.

EVALUATION OF HEART FAILURE

Exacerbations of heart failure have multiple potential causes; disease progression is just one of many possible reasons for worsening of dyspnea and other symptoms.

Disclosures: None.
Division of Cardiology, Saint Louis University School of Medicine, Saint Louis, MO, USA
* Corresponding author. Saint Louis University Hospital, 3635 Vista Avenue, 15th Floor, Saint Louis, MO 63110.
E-mail address: hauptmpj@slu.edu

Med Clin N Am 96 (2012) 943–954
http://dx.doi.org/10.1016/j.mcna.2012.07.004
0025-7125/12/$ – see front matter © 2012 Elsevier Inc. All rights reserved.

medical.theclinics.com

Box 1
Heart Failure Society of America working definition of heart failure

Heart failure is a syndrome caused by cardiac dysfunction, generally resulting from myocardial muscle dysfunction or loss and characterized by either left ventricular dilation or hypertrophy or both. Whether the dysfunction is primarily systolic or diastolic or mixed, it leads to neurohormonal and circulatory abnormalities, usually resulting in characteristic symptoms such as fluid retention, shortness of breath, and fatigue, especially on exertion. In the absence of appropriate therapeutic intervention, heart failure is usually progressive at the level of both cardiac function and clinical symptoms. The severity of clinical symptoms may vary substantially during the course of the disease process and may not correlate with changes in underlying cardiac function. Although heart failure is progressive and often fatal, patients can be stabilized and myocardial dysfunction and remodeling may improve, either spontaneously or as a consequence of therapy. In physiologic terms, heart failure is a syndrome characterized by either or both pulmonary and systemic venous congestion and/or inadequate peripheral oxygen delivery, at rest or during stress, caused by cardiac dysfunction.

From Heart Failure Society of America, Lindenfeld J, Albert NM, et al. HFSA 2010 comprehensive heart failure practice guideline. J Card Fail 2010;16:e1–94.

A brief list includes but is not limited to salt indiscretion, noncompliance with medications, new atrial arrhythmia, recent or concurrent myocardial ischemia, new onset of systemic illness such as infection, exacerbation of chronic obstructive pulmonary disease, new onset of thyroid disease or other metabolic abnormalities, and addition of new medications that contribute to sodium retention or negative inotropy. Nonphysiologic reasons are important and may be overlooked. As described by Amarasingham and colleagues,[2] multiple demographic and psychosocial factors can contribute to the worsening of clinical heart failure and subsequent readmission.

In the setting of a clinical deterioration, a careful accounting of symptoms is necessary to delineate if the patient is predominantly congested ("backward failure") or in a low-output state ("forward failure"), or both. Furthermore, symptoms can help the clinician decide whether the heart failure is predominantly right or left sided. The signs of heart failure are equally important to evaluate. One of the most fundamental parts of the physical examination is assessment of jugular venous pressure, which is a strong correlate of left atrial pressure in the absence of significant preexisting noncardiogenic pulmonary hypertension and/or severe tricuspid regurgitation.[3] Pulmonary rales, although often cited, are not sensitive in chronic or acute-on-chronic heart failure because of the capacity of the lung to increase venous capacitance and lymph drainage; by contrast, acute pulmonary edema with rales is generally seen in sudden-onset ischemic events or new catastrophic valvular abnormalities such as a ruptured papillary muscle. Classic signs of right-sided failure, such as ascites and lower extremity edema, should be noted. It is equally important to evaluate for the stigmata of peripheral hypoperfusion including a narrow pulse pressure, mental status changes such as inattention, and cool lower extremities in the absence of severe peripheral vascular disease.

Most imaging studies, blood chemistries, and biomarker values are supportive rather than diagnostic of an exacerbation of heart failure. Chest radiography can provide evidence for pulmonary congestion. Levels of brain natriuretic peptide (BNP) or N-terminal pro-BNP can help the clinician decide whether dyspnea is a result of heart failure or a noncardiac cause. However, for the patient with established heart failure and obvious signs of fluid overload, BNP elevation has more prognostic significance than immediate clinical relevance. An elevated creatinine level can reflect hypoperfusion to the kidney or elevated central venous pressure rather than intravascular volume depletion; elevated renal venous pressure is likely if jugular venous distention is also present. However, there is no noninvasive test, including echocardiography, that can definitively diagnose acute congestion or low cardiac output. Therefore, for the clinician, except for the use of a pulmonary artery catheter, accurate evaluation of the fluid and perfusion status of the patient using the history and physical examination remains the standard of care.[4]

THERAPEUTIC OPTIONS IN LOW CARDIAC OUTPUT SYNDROME

In those instances in which a low output state is suspected, the use of diuretic therapy alone may not suffice. Rather, selection of intravenous vasoactive therapy (either vasodilator or inotropic agent) may be required. It is important to highlight, however, that routine use of these agents, especially if the presentation is characterized by fluid overload rather than low output, is not recommended. Two important studies, OPTIME (The Outcomes of a Prospective Trial of Intravenous Milrinone for Exacerbations of Chronic Heart Failure) with milrinone and ASCEND-HF (Acute Study of Clinical Effectiveness of Nesiritide in Decompensated Heart Failure) with nesiritide, clearly demonstrated that a "one-size-fits-all" approach to heart failure exacerbations is not indicated.[5,6]

From a pathophysiologic standpoint, patients who have low output syndrome may have high end-diastolic pressures and markedly depressed intrinsic contractility that effectively impair the Frank-Starling mechanism. Further, with a limited forward output, a hemodynamic hierarchy comes into play so that the brain and heart vascular beds are vasodilated whereas other organs experience arterial vasoconstriction. Although an initial therapeutic goal remains the reduction of elevated filling pressures (if present), impaired cardiac output may limit the effectiveness of oral and intravenous loop diuretics. As noted, elevated central venous pressures may also lead to marked elevation of renal vein pressures, further impairing the responsiveness of the kidney to diuretic therapy and contributing to the development of cardiorenal syndrome.[7]

The administration of intravenous diuretics also activates neurohormonal responses, which can exacerbate vasoconstriction, limiting the natriuretic effect.[8] The DOSE (Diuretic Optimization Strategies Evaluation) study suggests that use of high-dose loop diuretics may lead to greater urine output in a conventional heart failure population but at a cost of an increased creatinine level.[9] Hence, in low-output states, characterized in part by a value of creatinine that may already be higher than baseline and/or increasing, diuretics will often fail to provide an adequate response.

Vasodilator therapy with intravenous sodium nitroprusside, nitroglycerin, or nesiritide may play a role in the management of fluid overload, especially in the setting of elevated systolic blood pressure or, in some instances, pulmonary hypertension. However, use of these agents may be limited by toxicity (nitroprusside), tachyphylaxis (nitroglycerin), and worsening renal function, especially at higher doses (nesiritide). The major limitation of nitroprusside is cyanide toxicity. Toxic side effects such as nausea and mental status changes are more likely to develop in patients receiving more than 250 µg/min for longer than 48 hours. Thiocyanate levels or methemoglobin measurement may not be available in timely fashion, although the development of a metabolic acidosis can be the earliest sign of toxicity; when present, suspected toxicity should be treated by discontinuation of the infusion. Tachyphylaxis can occur within hours of administration of high doses of nitroglycerin. Dilation of vessels by nitroglycerin is mediated through binding of heme to nitric oxide (NO) and activation of soluble guanylate cyclase (GC) in vascular smooth muscle, leading to the induction of the second-messenger cyclic guanosine monophosphate. Tachyphylaxis has traditionally been described as NO deficiency that attenuates GC activity as a result of tolerance and/or cross-tolerance to other nitrovasodilators. Recent studies have found that S-nitrosylation of soluble GC by endothelin-derived NO inhibits soluble GC activity, indicating aberrant NO bioactivity may also contribute to nitroglycerin tolerance.[10]

Nesiritide can significantly increase the risk of worsening renal function in patients with acute decompensated heart failure, especially with bolus administration and doses greater than 0.01 μg/kg/min.[11,12] Whether worsening renal function reflects hemodynamic effect or renal injury is unknown.[13] Despite these concerns, the use of vasodilators is reasonable in those situations where diuretics alone are not adequate to treat congestion and the patient may be exhibiting borderline cardiac output (based on signs and symptoms).

Inotropic therapy is a viable option in select patients when exacerbations of heart failure are punctuated by low cardiac output, end-organ hypoperfusion, and border-line blood pressure. Multiple mechanisms exist that regulate the basal contractile force of the myocardium, including length-dependent activation of cross-bridges, contraction frequency-dependent activation of contractile force, and catecholamine-induced inotropy. These mechanisms influence the force and velocity of contraction, and relaxation and energy consumption of the myocardium. The reader is referred to a classic text that helps define the elements involved in myocyte contraction and the abnormalities that occur in the setting of heart failure.[14] Unfortunately, most of the cellular or subcellular defects have been difficult to target with pharmacologic therapy in the acute setting, and the drugs themselves can have adverse pleiotropic effects, including worsening of the arrhythmic substrate.

The major inotropic agents are dopamine, dobutamine, and milrinone. The first 2 are β-adrenergic agonists and, as sympathomimetic agents have, in addition to direct effects on myocardial contractility, vascular and chronotropic effects. The third bypasses the β-receptor but, like the other agents, uses cyclic adenosine monophosphate (cAMP) as a secondary messenger. The relative value of these agents is debated, but in the β-blocker era, milrinone is the most likely to lead to a response at conventional doses.[15] The fact that milrinone is also more appropriately characterized as an inodilator, because of its vasodilatory effects on the pulmonary vasculature, adds to the strength of the argument in favor of its use. However, it is important to emphasize that patients who require inotropic therapy have a high short-term mortality rate. There are no well-designed placebo-controlled trials of intravenous inotropes versus placebo for chronic infusions, and trials with oral inotropes have frequently demonstrated poorer outcomes compared with placebo. In the REMATCH (Randomized Evaluation of Mechanical Assistance for the Treatment of Congestive Heart Failure) study, medically treated patients, of whom 72% were on intravenous inotrope, experienced a mortality rate of 100% at just over 2 years of follow-up.[16] In a Medicare cohort requiring chronic continuous intravenous inotrope infusions, mortality was 42.6% at 6 months.[17] Therefore, it is advisable to set realistic goals for inotropic therapy, with a focus on symptom relief.

DOPAMINE

For decades, dopamine has been known to stimulate β-adrenergic, α-adrenergic, and dopaminergic receptors in a dose-dependent fashion. Dopamine also induces the release of norepinephrine from sympathetic nerve terminals, but at low doses (1–3 μg/kg/min), it can cause renal and peripheral vasodilation. Intermediate infusion rates of 4 to 8 μg/kg/min also stimulate α- and β-adrenergic receptors in the vasculature and myocardium. The β-adrenergic stimulation results in positive inotropic and chronotropic actions, causing increased heart rate, stroke volume, and cardiac output. α-Adrenergic stimulation results in peripheral and venous constriction, which causes increased arterial pressure and increased cardiac filling pressure as a result of increased venous return to the heart. At higher infusion rates (>8 μg/kg/min), the α-adrenergic effect becomes predominant, resulting in more vasoconstriction.

The use of "renal dose" dopamine (1–3 μg/kg/min) has long been debated as an intervention to induce renal vasodilation and enhance renal function. A meta-analysis of low doses of dopamine given to reduce the incidence and severity of renal failure in critically ill patients revealed no improvement in rates of death or renal failure.[18] The overall clinical efficacy of dopamine's effect on diuresis is similar to that of dobutamine. The clinician must be aware of the risk of tachyarrhythmias and ischemia, which can be observed even with low doses.

DOBUTAMINE

Dobutamine is a sympathomimetic drug that exerts its effect through direct stimulation of $β_1$-receptors with little α-adrenergic effect, which leads to increased cardiac contractility and peripheral vasodilation and results in increased stroke volume, stroke work, and cardiac output. The major dose-limiting side effects are tachycardia and increased atrial and/or ventricular ectopy. These issues were highlighted in the PRECEDENT (Prospective Randomized Evaluation of Cardiac Ectopy with Dobutamine or Natrecor Therapy) study, which examined the safety of dobutamine compared with nesiritide. The study consisted of 255 patients randomized to receive intravenous nesiritide or dobutamine and assessed with 24-hour Holter monitoring before and during drug therapy. Dobutamine was associated with substantial proarrhythmic and chronotropic effects in patients with decompensated heart failure, whereas nesiritide actually reduced ventricular ectopy or had a neutral effect.[19] The investigators concluded that nesiritide may be a safer short-term treatment than dobutamine for patients with decompensated heart failure.

When dobutamine therapy is initiated, the lowest possible dose should be used to produce the desired effect. Increasing severity of hypoperfusion usually requires higher doses. There may be little benefit from increasing the dose to greater than 10 μg/kg/min, and other therapies should be considered as the dose approaches 15 μg/kg/min (**Table 1**). Tachyphylaxis is known to occur with prolonged infusions, and eosinophilic hypersensitivity including myocarditis has been reported in this setting,[20] although the clinical relevance of the latter finding is unclear.

MILRINONE

Milrinone is a phosphodiesterase (PDE) III inhibitor that prevents degradation of cAMP, thus increasing protein kinase A activity. Protein kinase A phosphorylation of calcium channels permits increased intracellular calcium influx, resulting in increased myocardial inotropy. As noted, milrinone auguments cardiac function independently of

Table 1 Inotrope dosing		
Inotrope	**Initial Dose (μg/kg/min)**	**Suggested Dose Range (μg/kg/min)**
Dopamine	1–2	1–15
Dobutamine	2.5–5	2.5–10
Milrinone	0.250	0.250–0.750[a]

Bolus infusions are generally not required or advised.
[a] Requires dose adjustment with impaired glomerular filtration rate.

β-adrenergic receptors. In general, administration does not require invasive hemodynamic monitoring. Initiation with a bolus is also discouraged to avoid an early hypotensive effect; by 30 minutes, the hemodynamic effects are not distinguishable between administrations by bolus followed by continuous infusion versus continuous infusion alone.[21] The formal recommendation for a starting dose is 0.25 to 0.75 μg/kg/min with dose adjustment in the presence of renal failure; the authors have found that doses as low as 0.125 μg/kg/min can be also effective.

In an elegant hemodynamic study by Colucci and colleagues[22] performed before the widespread use of β-blockers for heart failure, patients in the lowest baseline quartile of contractility responded better to milrinone than to dobutamine. The reason for this finding likely relates to the downregulation of β-receptors, which may be most significant in the patients with the most advanced heart failure. Because milrinone circumvents the β-receptor, it may be more effective than any catecholamine-based drug, including dobutamine. In an important study by Lowes and colleagues,[23] dobutamine produced an increase in cardiac index only at doses that are not typically used to treat heart failure (15–20 μg/kg/min) compared with conventional dosing with milrinone, when patients were chronically maintained on β-blockers. In addition, milrinone as a vasodilator can reduce right ventricular afterload, an important consideration if significant elevations of pulmonary arterial pressure or pulmonary vascular resistance are present. Another advantage over dobutamine is that tachyphylaxis is generally not observed.

However, the routine use of milrinone in the setting of decompensated heart failure is not indicated. In the OPTIME study, no benefit from milrinone treatment was observed in number of hospital days, other measurements of improvement in chronic heart failure, or the ability to institute oral drugs that improve long-term prognosis; by contrast, milrinone caused an increase in early adverse events related to hypotension and atrial arrhythmias.[5] Furthermore, intermittent scheduled infusions of intravenous inotropic agents for the chronic management of heart failure are not appropriate, because of the lack of convincing placebo-controlled data about both safety and efficacy (ie, reduction in hospitalizations); hence, it is a Class III recommendation according to American College of Cardiology/American Heart Association guidelines.[24]

OTHER INOTROPES

Multiple oral inotropes have failed in clinical trials, including vesnarinone, milrinone, pimobendan, enoximone, and flosequinan (**Table 2**).[25–29] Historically, the oral doses selected for the randomized clinical trials were based on interpretation of dose response in short-term invasive hemodynamic studies that demonstrated reductions in pulmonary capillary wedge pressure and increases in cardiac index. The lack of translation to longer-term benefit was unexpected. The reasons for the difference between effects on short-term surrogate end points and meaningful long-term clinical end points are not definitively known, but the list of possible explanations includes inappropriate (high) dosing, incorrect dosing interval, deleterious effects of large peak-to-trough differences in serum concentrations, adverse effects on heart rate, chronically increased metabolic demand and oxygen consumption, and proarrhythmia. It is conceivable that the presence of an implantable cardioverter-defibrillator (ICD) would have prevented premature sudden deaths precipitated by proarrhythmic effects of some oral inotropes, as most of the pivotal studies with oral inotropes were performed in the pre-ICD era; however, this remains an unproven hypothesis.

Table 2	
Inotropes that failed in clinical trials	
Inotrope	**Study**
Enoximone	EMOTE[28]
Flosequinan	PROFILE[29]
Levosimendan	REVIVE I, REVIVE II, SURVIVE[34,35]
Oral milrinone	PROMISE[27]
Pimobendan	PICO[26]
Vesnarinone	VEST[25]

Abbreviations: EMOTE, Enoximone in intravenous Inotrope-Dependent subjects; PICO, Pimobendan in Congestive Heart Failure; PROFILE, Prospective Randomized Flosequinan Longevity Evalution Investigators; PROMISE, Prospective Randomized Milrinone Survival Evaluation Study group; REVIVE I, Randomized multicentre Evaluation of intravenous Levosimendan efficacy versus placebo in short term treatment of decompensated heart failure; REVIVE II, Randomized multicentre Evaluation of intravenous Levosimendan efficacy versus placebo in the short term treatment of decompensated chronic heart failure; SURVIVE, Survival of patients with acute heart failure in need of intravenous inotropic support trial; VEST, Vesnarinone Trial investigators

Intravenous levosimendan, a calcium sensitizer, has been subjected to an extensive clinical development program. Levosimendan produces greater contractility by enhancing the binding of calcium to cardiac troponin C. Despite structural similarity with molecules belonging to the PDE-inhibitor family, levosimendan does not increase intracellular levels of cAMP or intracellular calcium. In fact, several reports have stated that levosimendan either did not increase the intracellular calcium at concentrations that are likely to occur in vivo or did not take it to levels high enough to explain its positive inotropic effect at therapeutic concentrations.[30] In addition to calcium sensitization, levosimendan also stimulates adenosine triphosphate (ATP)-sensitive K^+ channels that are suppressed by intracellular ATP. Finally, levosimendan opens the cardiac mitochondrial ATP-sensitive K^+ channels, a potentially cardioprotective mechanism linked to the preconditioning in response to oxidative stress.[31] However, despite these insights into mechanism of action and very intriguing early data from studies such as LIDO (Levosimendan Infusion versus Dobutamine) and CASINO (Calcium Sensitizer or Inotrope or None in Low Output Heart Failure),[32,33] the drug failed in larger, more definitive studies because of safety issues[34] or lack of efficacy.[35] The drug is approved for use in some European countries but not in the United States, and there is little indication that it or any other related drug will be able to meet the high regulatory bar set by the Food and Drug Administration.

INOTROPES UNDER INVESTIGATION

Omecamtiv mecarbil is a cardiac-specific myosin activator. Omecamtiv accelerates the rate-limiting step in actin-myosin cross-bridging through enhanced removal of phosphate from myosin, thus accelerating the transition of actin-myosin from a weakly bound to a strongly bound state. It also reduces ATP hydrolysis by inhibiting nonproductive phosphate release.[36] These cellular alterations result in increased left ventricular systolic ejection time, sarcomere shortening, and stroke volume without altering blood pressure or velocity of contraction.[37] At present, the drug is being studied in the ATOMIC-AHF (A Trial of Omecamtiv Mecarbil to Increase Contractility in Acute Heart Failure) trial.[38] However, unless the drug lowers the heart rate (preferably through a non–reflex-mediated mechanism), a prolongation of systole may not be advantageous unless it somehow also improves myocardial energetics.

USE OF INOTROPIC THERAPY TO BRIDGE TO β-BLOCKADE

In a small minority of patients with decompensated heart failure, the use of milrinone can be considered as a bridge to β-blockade.[39,40] However, in most cases, as demonstrated in the COPERNICUS (Carvedilol Prospective Randomized Cumulative Survival Study Group) study, patients with advanced heart failure tolerate initiation of β-blockers without the need for inotropic support as long as clinical euvolemia is present.[41]

BRIDGE TO TRANSPLANT OR VENTRICULAR ASSIST DEVICE

Continuous infusions of intravenous inotrope are frequently used in patients awaiting heart transplantation; the need for such agents elevates the patient on the transplant waiting list in the United States.[42] These patients are also often evaluated for placement of a left ventricular assist device as a bridge to transplant or destination therapy; in some cases, intravenous inotropes are continued after device placement to support the right ventricle. A similar approach is often taken in other heart failure surgeries, especially if right ventricular failure and/or pulmonary hypertension are present, which can limit left ventricular filling and reduce blood pressure. Given the pulmonary vasodilatory effects and the absence of tachyphylaxis, the authors prefer milrinone in these settings.

HOME INTRAVENOUS INOTROPIC THERAPY AND PALLIATION

The American College of Cardiology/American Heart Association guidelines state "continuous intravenous infusion of a positive inotropic agent may be considered for palliation of symptoms in patients with refractory end-stage heart failure" and categorize infusions as a Class IIb (level of evidence C) recommendation.[24] Consensus opinion supports this option as well, with the additional proviso that deactivation of the shock function of ICDs should be considered when inotropic therapy is selected.[43,44] The mortality rate in this patient cohort is high, but intravenous inotropes may also contribute to a reduction in hospital days, possibly mediated through improved symptoms.[17]

If chronic continuous inotropic therapy is under consideration for palliative management, right-sided heart catheterization may be necessary in most circumstances to document a hemodynamic response. According to regulations of the Centers for Medicare and Medicaid Services, a 20% increase in cardiac index or a 20% decrease in pulmonary capillary wedge pressure is required for reimbursement.[45,46] A clinical conundrum arises when a patient does not have baseline hemodynamic data available but has already been started on inotropic therapy to stabilize the condition. In these cases, despite the risk of deterioration, it is often necessary to completely stop the drug and obtain baseline hemodynamic measurements to document an improvement if indefinite continuous therapy is anticipated. Patients who receive this therapy are often candidates for hospice, but from a practical standpoint, 2 barriers exist. First, some hospice medical directors have a limited experience with heart failure and may view the use of intravenous inotropes as a "life-prolonging" treatment.[47] Second, the costs associated with infusions may exceed the per diem for hospice care.[48]

ORAL INOTROPES AND PALLIATION

An intriguing alternative to intravenous inotropic therapy for patients with terminal heart failure who are not candidates for transplantation, advanced surgical interventions, or experimental approaches is the use of oral agents in the inotrope class. Because survival is not the goal, the potentially negative effect on mortality may be a reasonable tradeoff in some patients to achieve improved symptoms. However, there is a paucity of data in this area, limited to small studies including one with oral levosimendan.[49]

CHALLENGES IN INOTROPIC DRUG DEVELOPMENT

Given the record of failure in this therapeutic area and the focus on safety, the pathway for regulatory approval for a novel inotrope is not straightforward. Even the definition and utility of acute end points remain uncertain.[50] The use of composite or combined end points is useful, but consensus has not been reached about the time points for efficacy and safety measurements. Given the high event rates of hospitalization, adverse events such as symptomatic arrhythmia, and mortality, these studies require fewer patients than those designed to evaluate the impact of interventions in chronic heart failure. The need for rescue with additional intravenous vasoactive therapy and/or mechanical support is a particularly appealing way to define worsening of heart failure, but these decisions are likely based on physician global assessment and are subject to variation by physician and site. Furthermore, there remains significant heterogeneity in the severity of illness among patients with decompensated heart failure. Nevertheless, an inotrope that does not increase heart rate, oxygen demand, or frequency and severity of arrhythmia could have a meaningful impact on the management of heart failure.

SUMMARY

Inotropic therapy remains an option in the management of patients with symptoms of advanced heart failure due to systolic dysfunction who do not respond to conventional therapies. The decision to use this class is largely predicated on an accurate evaluation of the patient's fluid and perfusion status. Selection of the appropriate agent and dosing regimens requires an understanding of the underlying pathophysiology of heart failure and concomitant therapy. Most important, the goals of care should be stated clearly, given inherent risks associated with this class of drug.

REFERENCES

1. Roger VL, Go AS, Lloyd-Jones DM, et al. Heart disease and stroke statistics—2011 update: a report from the American Heart Association. Circulation 2011;123:e18–209.
2. Amarasingham R, Moore BJ, Tabak YP, et al. An automated model to identify heart failure patients at risk for 30-day readmission or death using electronic medical record data. Med Care 2010;48:981–8.
3. Drazner MH, Rame JE, Stevenson LW, et al. Prognostic importance of elevated jugular venous pressure and a third heart sound in patient with heart failure. N Engl J Med 2001;345:574–81.
4. Heart Failure Society of America, Lindenfeld J, Albert NM, et al. HFSA 2010 Comprehensive heart failure practice guideline. J Card Fail 2010;16:e1–194.
5. Cuffe MS, Califf RM, Adams KF, et al. Short-term intravenous milrinone for acute exacerbation of chronic heart failure. JAMA 2002;287:1541–7.
6. O'Connor CM, Starling RC, Hernandez AF, et al. Effect of nesiritide in patients with acute decompensated heart failure. N Engl J Med 2011;365:32–43.
7. Metra M, Davison B, Bettari L, et al. Is worsening renal function an ominous prognostic sign in patients with acute heart failure? The role of congestion and its interaction with renal function. Circ Heart Fail 2012;5:54–62.

8. Francis GS, Siegel RM, Goldsmith SR, et al. Acute vasoconstrictor response to intravenous furosemide in patients with chronic congestive heart failure, activation of the neurohormonal axis. Ann Intern Med 1985;103:1–6.

9. Felker MG, Kerry LL, Bul DA, et al. Diuretic strategies in patients with acute decompensated heart failure. N Engl J Med 2011;364:797–805.

10. Sayed N, Kim DD, Fioramonti X, et al. Nitroglycerin-induced S-nitrosylation and desensitization of soluble guanylyl cyclase contribute to nitrate tolerance. Circ Res 2008;103:606–14.

11. Riter HG, Redfield MM, Burnett JC, et al. Nonhypotensive low-dose nesiritide has differential renal effects compared with standard-dose nesiritide in patients with acute decompensated heart failure and renal dysfunction. J Am Coll Cardiol 2006;47:2334–5.

12. Munger MA, Ng TM, Van Tassell BW. Controversy and conflict in the treatment of acute decompensated heart failure: nesiritide as evidence-based treatment. Pharmacotherapy 2007;27:619–25.

13. Sackner-Bernstein JD, Skopicki HA, Aaronson KD. Risk of worsening renal function with nesiritide in patients with acutely decompensated heart failure. Circulation 2005;111:1487–91.

14. Colucci WS. Positive inotropic/vasodilator agents. Cardiol Clin 1989;7:131–44.

15. Lowes BD, Tsvetkova T, Eichhorn EJ, et al. Milrinone versus dobutamine in heart failure subjects treated chronically with carvedilol. Int J Cardiol 2001;81:141–9.

16. Rose EA, Gelijns AC, Moskowitz AJ, et al. Randomized evaluation of mechanical assistance for the treatment of congestive heart failure (REMATCH) study group. N Engl J Med 2001;345:1435–43.

17. Hauptman PJ, Mikolajcak P, George A, et al. Chronic inotropic therapy in end-stage heart failure. Am Heart J 2006;152:1096 e1-1096 e8.

18. Friedrich JO, Adhikari N, Herridge MS, et al. Meta-analysis: low-dose dopamine increases urine output but does not prevent renal dysfunction or death. Ann Intern Med 2005;142:510–24.

19. Burger AJ, Horton DP, Lejemtel R, et al. Effect of nesiritide (B-type natriuretic peptide) and dobutamine on ventricular arrhythmias in the treatment of patients with acutely decompensated congestive heart failure: the PRECEDENT study. Am Heart J 2002;144:1102–8.

20. Takkenberg JJ, Czer LS, Fishbein MC, et al. Eosinophilic myocarditis in patients awaiting heart transplantation. Crit Care Med 2004;32:714–21.

21. Baruch L, Patacsil P, Hameed A, et al. Pharmacodynamic effects of milrinone with and without a bolus loading infusion. Am Heart J 2001;141:266–73.

22. Colucci WS, Wright RF, Jaski BE, et al. Milrinone and dobutamine in severe heart failure: differing hemodynamic effects and individual patient responsiveness. Circulation 1986;73:III175–83.

23. Lowes BD, Simon MA, Tsetkova TO, et al. Inotropes in the beta-blocker era. Clin Cardiol 2000;23(Suppl III):11–6.

24. Jessup M, Abraham WT, Casey DE, et al. 2009 Focused update: ACCF/AHA guidelines for the diagnosis and management of heart failure in adults: a report of the American College of Cardiology Foundation/American Heart Association Task Force on Practice Guidelines: developed in collaboration with the International Society for Heart and Lung Transplantation. Circulation 2009;119: 1977–2016.

25. Cohn JN, Goldstein SO, Greenberg BH, et al. A dose-dependent increase in mortality with vesnarinone among patients with severe heart failure. Vesnarinone trial investigators. N Engl J Med 1998;339:1810–6.

26. Lubsen J, Just H, Hjalmarsson AC, et al. Effect of pimobendan on exercise capacity in patients with heart failure: main results from the pimobendan in congestive heart failure (PICO) trial. Heart 1996;76:223–31.

27. Packer M, Carver JR, Rodeheffer RJ, et al. Effect of oral milrinone on mortality in severe chronic heart failure. The PROMISE study research group. N Engl J Med 1991;325:1468–75.

28. Feldman AM, Oren RM, Abraham WT, et al. Low-dose oral enoximone enhances the ability to wean patients with ultra-advanced heart failure from intravenous inotropic support: results of the oral enoximone in intravenous inotrope-dependent subjects trial. Am Heart J 2007;154:861–9.

29. Packer M, Rouleau J, Swedberg K, et al. Effect of flosequinan on survival in chronic heart failure: preliminary results of the PROFILE study [abstract]. Circulation 1993;88(Suppl I):301.

30. Szilagyi S, Pollesello P, Levijoki J, et al. Two inotropes with different mechanism of action: contractile, PDE inhibitory and direct myofibrillar effects of levosimendan and enoximone. J Cardiovasc Pharmacol 2005;46:369–76.

31. Hassenfuss G, Pieske B, Castell M, et al. Influence of the novel inotropic agent levosimendan on isometric tension and calcium cycling in failing human myocardium. Circulation 1998;98:2141–7.

32. Follath F, Cleland JG, Just H, et al. Efficacy and safety of intravenous levosimendan compared with dobutamine in severe low-output heart failure (the LIDO study): a randomised double-blind trial. Lancet 2002;360:196–202.

33. Cleland JGF, Ghosha J, Freemantle N, et al. Clinical trials update and cumulative meta-analyses from the American College of Cardiology: WATCH, SCD-HeFT, DINAMIT, CASINO, INSPIRE, STRATUS-US, RIO-Lipids and cardiac resynchronisation therapy in heart failure. Eur J Heart Fail 2004;6:501–8.

34. Cleland JG, Freemantle N, Coletta AP, et al. Clinical trials update from the American Heart Association: REPAIR-AMI, ASTAMI, JELIS, MEGA, REVIVE-II, SURVIVE, and PROACTIVE. Eur J Heart Fail 2006;8:105–10.

35. Mebazaa A, Nieminen MS, Packer M, et al. Levosimendan vs dobutamine for patients with acute decompensated heart failure. JAMA 2007;297:1883–91.

36. Malik FL, Morgan BP. Cardiac myosin activation, part 1: from concept to clinic. J Mol Cell Cardiol 2011;51:454–61.

37. Teerlink J. Dose-dependent augmentation of cardiac systolic function with the selective cardiac myosin activator, omecamtiv mecarbil: a first-in-man study. Lancet 2011;378:667–75.

38. Study to evaluate the safety and efficacy of IV infusion treatment with omecamtiv mecarbil in subjects with left ventricular systolic dysfunction hospitalized for acute heart failure. Available at: http://clinicaltrials.gov/ct2/show/NCT01300013?term=omecamtiv&recr=Open&cond=acute+heart+failure&rank=1. Accessed May 25, 2012.

39. Hauptman PJ, Woods D, Pritzker MR, et al. Novel use of a short-acting intravenous beta blocker in combination with inotropic therapy as a bridge to chronic oral beta blockade in patients with advanced heart failure. Clin Cardiol 2002;25:247–9.

40. Shakar SF, Abraham WT, Gilbert EM, et al. Combined oral positive inotropic and beta-blocker therapy for treatment of refractory class IV heart failure. J Am Coll Cardiol 1998;31:1336–40.

41. Packer M, Coats AJ, Fowler MD, et al. Effect of carvedilol on survival in severe chronic heart failure. N Engl J Med 2001;344:1651–8.

42. Allocation of thoracic organs. Available at: http://optn.transplant.hrsa.gov/PoliciesandBylaws2/policies/pdfs/Policy_9.pdf. Accessed May 25, 2012.

43. Goodlin SJ, Hauptman PJ, Arnold R, et al. Consensus statement: palliative and supportive care in advanced heart failure. J Card Fail 2004;10:200–9.
44. Allen LA, Stevenson LW, Grady KL, et al. Decision making in advanced heart failure: a scientific statement from the American Heart Association. Circulation 2012;125:1928–52.
45. Home parenteral inotropic therapy: data collection form. Available at: https://coverage.cms.fu.com/lcd_area/lcd_uploads/5044_15/HomeParenteralInotropicTherapyDataCollectionForm.pdf. Accessed August 9, 2012.
46. DMERC Medicare advisory. Available at: http://www.cgsmedicare.com/jc/pubs/adv/pdf/1995/December%201995.pdf. Accessed May 25, 2012.
47. Kutner J, Goodlin SJ, Connor SR, et al. Hospice care for heart failure patients. J Pain Symptom Manage 2005;29:525–8.
48. Rich MW, Shore BL. Dobutamine for patients with end-stage heart failure in a hospice program? J Palliat Med 2003;6(1):93–7.
49. Nieminen MS, Cleland JG, Eha J, et al. Oral levosimendan in patients with severe chronic heart failure—the PERSIST study. Eur J Heart Fail 2008;10:1246–54.
50. Packer M. Proposal for a new clinical end point to evaluate the efficacy of drugs and devices in the treatment of chronic heart failure. J Card Fail 2001;7:176–82.

Renal Dysfunction in Heart Failure

Robert T. Cole, MD[a,*], Amirali Masoumi, MD[a],
Filippos Triposkiadis, MD[b], Gregory Giamouzis, MD[b],
Vasiliki Georgiopoulou, MD[a], Andreas Kalogeropoulos, MD, PhD[a],
Javed Butler, MD, MPH[a]

KEYWORDS

- Chronic kidney disease • Heart failure • Worsening renal function
- Cardiorenal syndrome

KEY POINTS

- Both chronic kidney disease and worsening renal function are associated with worse outcomes, but our understanding of the complex bidirectional interactions between the heart and kidney remains poor.
- When addressing these interactions, one must consider the impact of intrinsic renal disease resulting from medical comorbidities on outcomes of patients with heart failure.
- Worsening renal function in heart failure is the result of a complex, multifactorial process that includes: RAAS and SNS activation, hemodynamic aberrations, pharmacological interventions, and inflammation/cytokine activation..
- The development of novel renal biomarkers will enable earlier detection of WRF and someday allow for the administration of reno-protective strategies.

INTRODUCTION

Renal dysfunction is common in patients with heart failure (HF), with a prevalence ranging from 20% to 57% in patients with chronic, stable HF[1-9] and 30% to 67% in large registries of patients admitted with acutely decompensated HF (ADHF).[10-12] In addition, worsening renal function (WRF) occurs in 18% to 40% of patients during hospitalization for ADHF,[13-19] an important subset of patients with generally guarded prognosis. The interplay between the heart and the kidney in patients with HF is a complex relationship, and a complete understanding of the bidirectional interactions between these 2 organs remains elusive. While attempts have been made to better define and categorize these interactions, to date these definitions lack clinical utility. In its simplest form, the so-called cardiorenal syndrome (CRS) has been described as a complex disorder of the heart and kidneys whereby acute or chronic dysfunction in one organ may result in acute or

Conflict of interest: None.
Funding sources: None.
[a] Emory University, Atlanta, GA, USA; [b] Larissa University Hospital, Larissa, Greece
* Corresponding author. Emory University Hospital, Center for Heart Failure Therapy, 1365 Clifton Road Northeast, Suite AT 430, Atlanta, GA 30322.
E-mail address: rtcole@emory.edu

Med Clin N Am 96 (2012) 955–974
http://dx.doi.org/10.1016/j.mcna.2012.07.005
0025-7125/12/$ – see front matter © 2012 Elsevier Inc. All rights reserved.

medical.theclinics.com

chronic dysfunction in the other.[20] The syndrome has been further broken down into 1 of 5 categories, based on the acute or chronic nature of the disease course and whether or not the primary precipitant of dysfunction is the heart, the kidney, or a third independent process affecting both the heart and kidneys (**Table 1**).[20]

Yet such categorization does little to shed light on the underlying pathophysiology of the CRS as it pertains to the patient with HF. In truth, many factors must be considered in the development of a comprehensive construct of renal dysfunction in HF. One must first consider the importance of intrinsic renal disease and the adverse effects of common medical comorbidities on kidney function in HF patients. Diabetes mellitus, hypertension, and renovascular disease are common in the HF population, and can lead to significant intrinsic, chronic kidney disease (CKD). Next, it is important to recognize the significance of WRF in HF and the many factors that can predispose to it, including: (1) the deleterious acute and chronic effects of activation of the renin-angiotensin-aldosterone system (RAAS) and sympathetic nervous system (SNS), (2) the direct effects of hemodynamic aberrations, (3) the effects of pharmacologic interventions (eg, diuretics, angiotensin-converting enzyme [ACE] inhibitors), and (4) the role of inflammation and cytokine activation. All of these factors likely play critical roles to varying degrees in the individual HF patient, perhaps accounting for the heterogeneous presentations of patients with WRF in HF. Although the pathophysiology may not be entirely clear, most HF patients with CKD or WRF have a worse prognosis than those without renal involvement.[9,13,16,21–27] In the near future, the development of novel biomarkers of renal dysfunction may enable earlier and more accurate detection of renal damage in HF, and pave the way for the administration of future renoprotective strategies.

Table 1 Cardiorenal syndrome (CRS) subtypes		
Cardiorenal Subtype	**Description**	**Examples/Etiology**
CRS Type 1 (acute CRS)	Rapid worsening of cardiac function leading to acute kidney injury	Acute MI with cardiogenic shock, ADSHF, acute valvular insufficiency
CRS Type 2 (chronic CRS)	Chronic abnormalities in cardiac function leading to chronic kidney disease	Chronic inflammation, long-term RAAS and SNS activation, chronic hypoperfusion
CRS Type 3 (acute renocardiac syndrome)	Acute worsening of renal function leading to cardiac dysfunction (HF, arrhythmia, and so forth)	Uremia causing impaired contractility, hyperkalemia causing arrhythmias, volume overload causing pulmonary edema
CRS Type 4 (chronic renocardiac syndrome)	Chronic worsening of renal function leading to worsening cardiac function	CKD leading to LVH, coronary disease and calcification, diastolic dysfunction, and so forth
CRS Type 5	Acute or chronic systemic disease leading to both cardiac and renal dysfunction	Diabetes mellitus, amyloidosis, sepsis, vasculitis

Abbreviations: ADSHF, acute decompensated systolic heart failure; CKD, chronic kidney disease; HF, heart failure; LVH, left ventricular hypertrophy; MI, myocardial infarction; RAAS, renin-angiotensin-aldosterone system; SNS, sympathetic nervous system.

CHRONIC KIDNEY DISEASE IN HEART FAILURE
Definition

To fully understand the potential adverse effects of CKD in HF, one must first define CKD. According to the National Kidney Foundation (NKF) practice guidelines, glomerular filtration rate (GFR) is the best measure of renal function.[28] Of importance, the NKF practice guidelines do not recommend the use of serum creatinine (sCr) concentration as the sole measure of renal function,[28] as this value can be greatly affected by an individual's age, sex, race, muscle mass, and diet. Direct assessment of GFR requires measuring the renal clearance of a nontoxic exogenous marker such as inulin, which is freely filtered without any tubular secretion or reabsorption. Unfortunately, such a method is cumbersome and impractical for use in routine clinical practice. In lieu of directly measuring GFR, several formulas have been developed that reliably estimate GFR with relative accuracy. Of note, all of these formulas incorporate the sCr and some combination of age, sex, body size, and race, all factors that affect GFR to varying degrees. The formulas most frequently used in clinical practice include the Cockcroft-Gault (C-G),[29] Modification of Diet in Renal Disease (MDRD),[30] and Chronic Kidney Disease Epidemiology Collaboration (CKD-EPI)[31] equations (**Table 2**). Based on the estimated GFR (eGFR), individual patients can be classified into 1 of 5 categories of CKD (**Table 3**).

It is important to understand potential pitfalls in the various formulas for GFR, especially as they pertain to the HF population. Although the equations for estimating GFR are all relatively similar, the MDRD may be more precise in patients with lower GFR,[32] whereas the C-G equation is more precise in those with milder forms of CKD.[29] Unfortunately, both the MDRD and C-G formulas may misclassify the degree of CKD in up to 30% of patients and may be off by as much as 13.5 mL/min and 15.1 mL/min in their GFR estimations, respectively.[32] Of importance, all of these formulas tend to overestimate GFR in the setting of severe renal disease.[33,34] Finally, the MDRD equation was derived from a relatively young population (mean age 50 ± 12 years) with established CKD and excluded older patients.[30] It therefore may be inaccurate in the HF population, which comprises mostly patients older than 65 years.[35,36]

Table 2
Clinically used formulas for estimating glomerular filtration rate (GFR)

	Equation/Formula
Cockcroft-Gault (mL/min)	Male: $[(140 - \text{age}) \times (\text{weight})]/72 \times \text{sCr}$ Female: GFR $\times$ 0.85 BSA corrected: $\text{GFR}_{cg} \times (1.73/\text{BSA})$ (= mL/min/1.73 m^2)
MDRD (mL/min/1.73 m^2)	Male: $170 \times (\text{sCr})^{-0.999} \times (\text{age})^{-0.176} \times (\text{sU})^{-0.170} \times (\text{sAlb})^{+0.318}$ Black male: MDRD $\times$ 1.180 Female: MDRD $\times$ 0.76 Black female: MDRD $\times$ 0.762 $\times$ 1.180
CKD-EPI (mL/min/1.73 m^2)	Male: $141 \times \text{minimum} (\text{sCr}/0.9, 1)^{-0.411} \times \text{max} (\text{sCr}/0.9, 1)^{-1.209}$ $\times 0.993^{\text{Age}}$ Black male: CKD-EPI $\times$ 1.159 Female: $141 \times \text{minimum} (\text{sCr}/0.7, 1)^{-0.329} \times \text{max} (\text{sCr}/0.7, 1)^{-1.209}$ $\times 0.993^{\text{Age}} \times 1.018$ Black female: CKD-EPI (female) $\times$ 1.159

Abbreviations: BSA, body surface area; CKD-EPI, Chronic Kidney Disease Epidemiology Collaboration; MDRD, Modification of Diet in Renal Diseases; Alb, serum albumin; sCr, serum creatinine; sU, serum uric acid.

Table 3
Stages of chronic kidney disease (CKD)

CKD Stage	Description	GFR (mL/min/1.73 m^2)
Stage 1	Kidney damage with preserved GFR	$\geq$90
Stage 2	Kidney damage with mildly decreased GFR	60–89
Stage 3	Moderately reduced GFR	30–59
Stage 4	Severely reduced GFR	15–29
Stage 5	Kidney failure/end-stage renal disease	<15 (or dialysis)

Epidemiology and Prognosis

Retrospective analysis of several clinical trials has shown that the prevalence of CKD ranges between 20% and 57% in chronic, stable HF populations.[3–9] Of importance, many of these analyses included only patients with at least moderate renal dysfunction, defined as an eGFR of less than 60 mL/min (CKD stage III). Therefore patients with milder forms of CKD may not have been included, and represent a large population at risk for worse outcomes. A meta-analysis of 16 studies and more than 80,000 patients revealed that approximately 51% of outpatients with HF have some degree of renal dysfunction (eGFR <90 mL/min, sCr >1.0 mg/dL).[25]

While HF pathophysiology may contribute to the development of CKD, concomitant comorbidities also play an important role. For example, data from the Framingham Heart Study show that nearly 60% of patients with newly diagnosed HF had preexisting hypertension (HTN), and 25% were being treated for diabetes mellitus at the time of diagnosis, both important risk factors for CKD.[37] In addition, the median age at time of HF diagnosis was 78 years. It is known that GFR decreases by as much as 0.75 mL/min annually after the age of 30 years,[38,39] and this decline may accelerate in the elderly.[40] Finally, the presence of atheromatous renovascular disease (ARD) is increasingly recognized as a cause of renal dysfunction,[41] and ARD is reported to account for 15% of end-stage renal disease (ESRD) in the elderly.[42,43] One analysis found that 30% of HF patients have some degree of ARD when assessed by angiography.[44] ARD is therefore likely an important, often overlooked, source of renal dysfunction in HF.

Whatever the cause of CKD in HF, its presence is associated with a worse prognosis and poor outcomes. A retrospective cohort study of more than 600 recently discharged HF patients revealed that the presence of CKD (sCr >1.5 mg/dL in men, >1.4 mg/dL in women) was associated with a 43% increase in the relative risk of death.[26] Similarly, a large meta-analysis showed that any degree of renal dysfunction (eGFR <90 mL/min) was associated with a 48% increase in the relative risk of death[25]; those with moderate to severe renal dysfunction had an 81% increased risk. Many other studies have shown similarly poor survival in HF patients with CKD[4,9,27] as well as higher rates of readmission for HF.[45–49]

WORSENING RENAL FUNCTION IN HEART FAILURE
Definition, Epidemiology, and Prognosis

WRF in HF is common in patients with ADHF and complicates 18% to 40% of admissions.[13–19] Despite the association between WRF and worse clinical outcomes, a standard definition has not been adopted. The most commonly used definition in most studies is an increase in the sCr of greater than 0.3 mg/dL,[11,13,14,50,51] but others use a value of greater than 0.5 mg/dL,[15,21] greater than 0.2 mg/dL,[19] or a decrease in eGFR by 25%.[16] Regardless of the definition, development of WRF during hospitalization for ADHF is associated with poor outcomes in most, but not all studies. Several studies have shown that WRF is associated with an increased risk of in-hospital mortality and prolonged length of stay.[11,14,15,21,52] Krumholz and colleagues[17] found that an increase in sCr by greater than 0.3 mg/dL resulted in an increase in length of stay by 2.3 days, an increase in the cost by $1758, and an increase in in-hospital mortality odds by 2.72 times. Other studies have also shown that even minimal changes in renal function (increased sCr >0.1 mg/dL) are associated with worse outcomes,[15,25] although greater degrees of WRF result in higher rates of death.[19] WRF is also associated with postdischarge mortality, including reductions in 60-day[16] and 1-year survival.[18] However, Nohria and colleagues[50] did not find a correlation between WRF and outcomes in the ESCAPE (Evaluation Study of Congestive Heart Failure and Pulmonary Artery Catheterization Effectiveness) trial. Instead, they found that admission and discharge renal dysfunction better predicted mortality and rehospitalization.

Many investigators have attempted to identify risk factors for the development of WRF in HF. Several risk factors have been identified to date, including the presence of baseline renal dysfunction (admission sCr),[13,14,17,21,53] diabetes mellitus,[14,21,53] hypertension,[14,17,53] pulmonary edema,[13,17] low serum sodium,[21] male gender,[17] diastolic dysfunction by echocardiography,[21] and the presence of atrial fibrillation.[13] Although these factors may predispose patients to the development of WRF, they do little to shed light on the etiology of the disease process. In truth, the etiology of WRF is a complex, multifactorial process that is incompletely understood (**Fig. 1**).

Role of Neurohormonal Activation in Worsening Renal Function

The kidney plays a fundamental role in the adaptive responses in HF. As a response to renal underperfusion, the activation of the RAAS initially maintains circulating blood volume (by increasing sodium reabsorption) as well as GFR (through angiotensin II–mediated renal efferent arteriolar constriction).[54,55] However, prolonged RAAS activation leads to volume overload, congestion, worsening HF, cardiac fibrosis, and

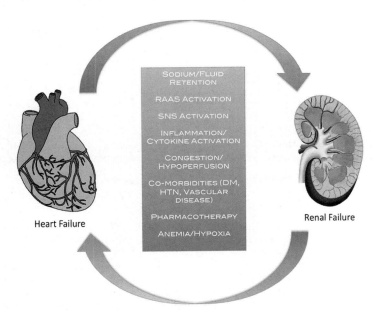

SODIUM/FLUID RETENTION

RAAS ACTIVATION

SNS ACTIVATION

INFLAMMATION/ CYTOKINE ACTIVATION

CONGESTION/ HYPOPERFUSION

CO-MORBIDITIES (DM, HTN, VASCULAR DISEASE)

PHARMACOTHERAPY

ANEMIA/HYPOXIA

Heart Failure

Renal Failure

Fig. 1. The complex bidirectional relationship between heart failure and renal disease.

adverse myocardial remodeling.[56–60] RAAS inhibition is therefore the cornerstone of long-term HF therapy. In addition to the harmful effects of RAAS activation on the heart, there is significant evidence that angiotensin II leads to progressive fibrosis of the kidney by activating fibroblasts and increasing extracellular matrix deposition, and through its effects as a proinflammatory cytokine (**Fig. 2**).[61] The use of agents that antagonize RAAS activation can prevent fibrosis and inflammatory cell infiltration[62–64] and prevent WRF.

The SNS is closely linked to RAAS activation in the kidneys and plays a significant role in renal physiology. Renal dysfunction, like HF, is associated with sympathetic overactivity, and the level of activity is an independent predictor of death in patients with CKD.[65,66] The renal sympathetic nerves modulate many functions of the kidney through their innervation of the tubules, the afferent and efferent vessels, and the juxtaglomerular granular cells.[67] Sympathetic overactivity as found in HF and CKD ultimately leads to WRF through multiple mechanisms. The stimulation of α1-adrenergic receptors in vascular smooth muscle results in increased renal vascular resistance[68] and preferential efferent arteriolar constriction, thus serving to increase the filtration fraction at the expense of renal blood flow.[69] Stimulation of β1-adrenergic receptors of the juxtaglomerular cells results in the release of renin[70] and therefore

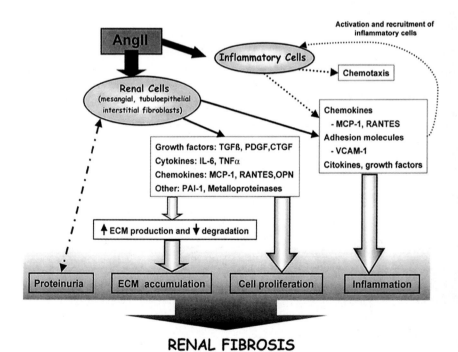

RENAL FIBROSIS

Fig. 2. The pathophysiology of angiotensin II and renal fibrosis. Angiotensin II leads to renal fibrosis through direct effects on renal cells and through activation of inflammation. CTGF, connective tissue growth factor; ECM, extracellular matrix; IL, interleukin; MCP, monocyte chemotactic protein; OPN, osteopontin; PAI, plasminogen activator inhibitor; PDGF, platelet-derived growth factor; RANTES, regulated upon activation, normal T-cell expressed, and secreted; TGF, transforming growth factor; TNF, tumor necrosis factor; VCAM, vascular cell adhesion molecule. (*Reprinted from* Mezzano SA, Ruiz-Ortega M, Egido J. Angiotensin II and renal fibrosis. Hypertension 2001;38:635–8.)

downstream RAAS activation, further worsening both HF and WRF. Of importance, the use of carvedilol (α1/β1-receptor blocker) has been shown to reduce renal vascular resistance, increase renal blood flow, and decrease tubular atrophy and interstitial fibrosis.[71] Considering these data, it is clear that the fundamental pathophysiology leading to progressive HF, RAAS and SNS activation, is also a cause of WRF, and highlights the importance of the bidirectional relationship of these 2 organs.

Hemodynamics and Worsening Renal Function

The historical concept that WRF in ADHF is a direct result of reduced cardiac output and "underperfusion" is an oversimplification. Several reports have failed to show a correlation between lower ejection fraction (EF) and WRF.[10,72–74] While reduction in cardiac output may play a role in WRF, especially at extremes,[75] the pathophysiology is more complex. The maintenance of an adequate renal perfusion pressure (RPP) is certainly affected by alterations in forward flow, but recent data suggest that alterations in congestive forces (central venous pressure, intra-abdominal pressure, and therefore elevated renal vein pressure) may play a more critical hemodynamic role in WRF.[76–79] Mullens and colleagues[78] reported that the 2 strongest predictors of WRF were a higher CVP on admission (18 $\pm$ 7 mm Hg vs 12 $\pm$ 6 mm Hg, P <.001) and a higher CVP after therapy (11 $\pm$ 8 mm Hg vs 8 $\pm$ 5 mm Hg, P <.04). Of note, there was no difference in cardiac index (CI) in patients with or without WRF, suggesting that lower CI did not play a role in WRF in this population. In a report of less-sick HF patients, Guglin and colleagues[79] showed that elevated CVP is associated with higher sCr and lower GFR, whereas there was no association between CI and renal function. In a heterogeneous population of patients undergoing right heart catheterization, higher CVP was associated with WRF as well as mortality.[77] Of interest, the relationship between CVP and estimated GFR was most pronounced in those patients with normal CI, again suggesting that congestive forces play a more critical role in the development of WRF.

Elevation in intra-abdominal pressure (IAP), as may be seen in a variety of surgical emergencies and the abdominal compartment syndrome, has been linked to WRF.[51,52] Considering that many patients with ADHF have significant visceral edema and ascites, it is feasible to hypothesize that they may have significant elevations in IAP and therefore impaired renal function. Mullens and colleagues[76] measured IAP in a cohort of patients with ADHF requiring right heart catheterization and tailored therapy, and showed a high prevalence of elevated IAP (>8 mm Hg) that was associated with worse renal function (**Fig. 3**). In addition, reductions in IAP with therapy were associated with improvements in renal function. There was no correlation with improvement in renal function and other hemodynamic variables.

Not all studies support the role of hemodynamic alterations as a cause of WRF in ADHF. Data from the ESCAPE trial showed no correlation between baseline hemodynamics or changes in hemodynamics during hospitalization and WRF.[50] Similarly, Testani and colleagues[80] found no difference in baseline, final, or change in hemodynamics when comparing patients with WRF during hospitalization and those with improved renal function (IRF) during hospitalization. Of note, both sets of patients (WRF and IRF) had worse outcomes than those with stable renal function.

Role of Pharmacotherapy in Worsening Renal Function

Diuretic therapy

Congestion is the hallmark of HF[81] and diuretics remain the mainstay of therapy. Despite their role, diuretics have not been proved to improve outcomes in randomized controlled trials. In fact, some data suggest that use of loop diuretics is associated with

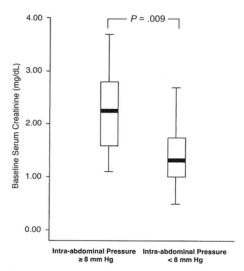

Fig. 3. Serum creatinine and intra-abdominal pressure. Patients admitted with intra-abdominal pressure greater than 8 mm Hg had higher creatinine levels on admission for acutely decompensated heart failure. (*Reprinted from* Mullens W, Abrahams Z, Skouri HN, et al. Elevated intra-abdominal pressure in acute decompensated heart failure: a potential contributor to worsening renal function? J Am Coll Cardiol 2008;51:300–6.)

increased risk of arrhythmic death,[82] hospitalization,[83] and long-term mortality.[83–85] These adverse effects are thought to result from secondary neurohormonal activation[86] and diuretic-induced electrolyte depletion.[82] In addition, escalating doses of loop diuretics in patients with ADHF has been linked to WRF. In a nested case-control study of 382 ADHF patients, Butler and colleagues[53] showed that higher doses of loop diuretics were associated with an increased risk of WRF independent of the amount of fluid loss. Similarly, in another study of 318 patients with ADHF, daily furosemide dose was a predictor of WRF and subsequent poor prognosis.[87] Hasselblad and colleagues[88] reviewed data from the ESCAPE trial and also found that higher diuretic dose (especially >300 mg/d) was an independent risk factor for mortality after adjusting for several variables. Of note, however, they did not find a significant correlation between change in sCr and maximal diuretic dose. The mechanisms whereby diuretics precipitate WRF are likely more complex than simple depletion of circulating volume. By increasing the sodium load to the distal tubule, diuretics may precipitate increases in the release of adenosine from the juxtaglomerular cells. Elevations in intrarenal adenosine in turn may lead to increased sodium reabsorption in the proximal tubule and constriction of the renal afferent arteriole, which reduces GFR.[89]

While it is clear that many patients requiring higher doses of diuretics during hospitalization for ADHF have an increased risk of WRF and therefore a worse prognosis, it is not clear if higher doses or WRF are a cause of worse outcomes. These patients may simply represent a subset of more advanced disease. To further complicate the picture, there are data to suggest that aggressive diuresis that results in WRF is associated with improved survival.[90] A retrospective analysis of the ESCAPE trial showed that aggressive diuresis resulting in hemoconcentration was associated with WRF; however, these patients had lower mortality at 180 days (**Fig. 4**).[90] Also, in the recent DOSE (Diuretic Optimization Strategies Evaluation) trial assessing optimal loop diuretic dosing strategies, higher bolus doses of diuretics were associated with

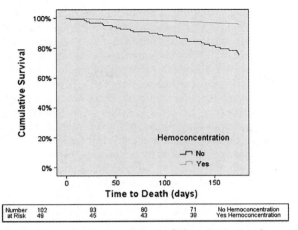

Fig. 4. Hemoconcentration and outcomes in heart failure. Patients who experienced hemo-concentration after dieresis had better long-term survival after discharge. (*Reprinted from* Testani JM, Chen J, McCauley BD, et al. Potential effects of aggressive decongestion during the treatment of decompensated heart failure on renal function and survival. Circulation 2010;122:265–2.)

greater diuresis, greater weight loss, improvement in dyspnea, and fewer serious adverse events compared with lower bolus doses, despite higher rates of transient WRF.[91] This transient WRF resolved by discharge and there was no difference in renal function at 60 days. Thus, in these 2 studies aggressive diuresis resulting in transient WRF was associated with improved outcomes.

ACE inhibition

ACE inhibition is a key component of HF therapy. The use of these agents results in reduced mortality, improved symptoms, and reduction in HF hospitalizations.[1,2,92] Use of ACE inhibitors is associated with an expected increase in sCr of up to 30%, especially in patients with a baseline sCr greater than 1.4 mg/dL.[93] This increase is the physiologic result of renal efferent arteriole dilation and subsequent decrease in GFR, and the value usually stabilizes within the first 2 months of treatment.[93] The continuation of ACE inhibition in these patients leads to long-term preservation of renal function, likely a result of inhibiting the proinflammatory and profibrotic effects of angiotensin II on the kidney.[62–64,94] Unfortunately, many patients are taken off this essential therapy in response to increases in sCr, despite their well-documented long-term benefits. Not all patients started on ACE inhibitors experience an increase in sCr, and an improvement in sCr in 24% of patients with ACE-inhibitor therapy has been reported.[95] There is clearly a subset of patients with HF who have difficulty tolerating ACE inhibition, including those with low blood pressure, higher doses of diuretics, volume contraction, and hyponatremia.[95,96] These patients may be more dependent on neurohormonal activation to maintain renal perfusion, and the inhibition of angiotensin II may result in marked WRF and hypotension.[97] Strategies to combat this issue include reduction in diuretic dose, reduction in ACE-inhibitor dose, or discontinuation of ACE inhibitors altogether in a few cases.[97]

Role of Inflammation

HF is associated with the activation of systemic inflammation and the upregulation of several inflammatory cytokines.[98] Of importance, these biomarkers correlate with HF severity and poor outcomes. For example, tumor necrosis factor α (TNF-α) and interleukin (IL)-6 levels are increased in HF, and are associated with increased mortality and worsening New York Heart Association class.[99–101] Elevated C-reactive protein (CRP) levels independently predict death[102,103] and readmission for worsening HF.[103] There are several theories as to why HF is associated with inflammation, including: (1) RAAS activation and direct angiotensin II–induced expression of TNF-α and IL-6[94,104,105]; (2) SNS activation leading to β-adrenergic–induced expression of inflammatory cytokines[106,107]; (3) venous congestion leading to endothelial activation and release of proinflammatory mediators[108,109]; and (4) venous congestion leading to translocation of intestinal gram-negative endotoxin (lipopolysaccharide) and resultant imflammation.[110–112] Circulating cytokines lead to the infiltration of inflammatory cells into the renal interstitium, resulting in tubular injury, fibrosis, and WRF.[98,113–115] Both TNF-α and IL-1 induce production of free radicals in the mesangial cells,[116] which can result in significant glomerular damage. In addition, both TNF-α and reactive oxygen species have been shown to inhibit renal sodium excretion and lead to worsening volume expansion,[117,118] which then causes further activation of SNS[67,119] and RAAS.[120,121]

MARKERS OF RENAL FUNCTION AND INJURY

As previously discussed, sCr levels are affected by muscle mass, which can be substantially reduced in the setting of cardiac cachexia. To combat this, many formulas (MDRD, C-G, CKD-EPI) have been developed to account for body size, age, and gender, among other variables. However, these formulas only estimate the ability of the kidney to filter the blood; they do not assess glomerular permeability, tubular function, or other actions of the kidney such as erythropoietin and production of vitamin D.[122] In addition, these measures are slow to detect kidney injury and may lag injury by several days, making them clinically less useful. Newer serum and urinary biomarkers may offer advantages over sCr and sCr-based formulas to detect WRF and renal injury in HF, and may provide this information in a timely manner (**Table 4**).

Blood Urea Nitrogen

Blood urea nitrogen (BUN) has long been measured clinically, but only recently has its correlation with HF prognosis been recognized. In the ADHERE registry, BUN was the best predictor of in-hospital mortality (BUN ≥43 mg/dL).[123] In another study, BUN remained the most sensitive predictor of 1-year mortality.[124] Finally, a retrospective study of the OPTIME-HF registry showed that changes in BUN during hospitalization are an independent predictor of 60-day mortality (BUN increase of 10 mg/dL over baseline).[16] While BUN levels are affected by changes in renal function, they are also influenced by dietary protein intake, catabolism, and tubular reabsorption. Therefore, despite its potential for use as a prognostic marker, BUN is an inaccurate marker of true renal function.

Cystatin C

Cystatin C is a low molecular weight protein produced by all nucleated cells.[125] It is freely filtered in the glomerulus, completely reabsorbed, and degraded in the tubules.[126] Cystatin C is unaffected by muscle mass or turnover, and therefore is an ideal measure of glomerular filtration.[126,127] It is a more reliable predictor of GFR than sCr,[128,129] although this has not been assessed in HF. In ADHF, cystatin C levels were an independent predictor of mortality, even in the presence of normal sCr.[130]

Table 4
Beyond serum creatinine and estimated GFR: biomarkers of renal dysfunction

Marker	Pros and Cons
BUN	PRO: Correlates well with prognosis, inexpensive, and easy to measure CON: Greatly affected by protein intake, catabolism, and tubular reabsorption → poor measure of true renal function
Cystatin C	PRO: excellent marker of GFR (better than sCr); not affected by intake, catabolism, and so forth; good marker of prognosis in CHF CON: more costly than sCr; clinicians unfamiliar with use and normals/abnormals
NGAL	PRO: excellent sensitivity and specificity to detect AKI; levels increase >24 h before sCr increases in response to injury CON: Plasma NGAL levels increase in settings of inflammation, making them less specific than urinary NGAL levels
KIM-1	PRO: Levels are elevated even with minimal GFR reductions; associated with death or HF hospitalization independent of GFR; increases 24 h before sCr in response to renal injury CON: Very few studies in HF at this time
NAG	PRO: Excellent predictor of AKI; levels are elevated even in the setting of minimally reduced GFR; associated with risk of death or HF hospitalization CON: Very few studies in HF at this time
FABP	PRO: Presence in the urine is sensitive and specific for AKI and predicts the need for renal replacement therapy and death CON: No data on ability to predict WRF in CHF
Albuminuria	PRO: Inexpensive, easy to measure; correlates with worse prognosis in HF CON: can be found in other disease states (DM, HTN), therefore low specificity

Abbreviations: AKI, acute kidney injury; BUN, blood urea nitrogen; DM, diabetes mellitus; FABP, fatty acid–binding protein; HTN, hypertension; KIM-1, kidney injury molecule 1; NAG, *N*-acetyl-β-D-glucosaminidase; NGAL, neutrophil gelatinase-associated lipocalin.

Neutrophil Gelatinase-Associated Lipocalin

Neutrophil gelatinase-associated lipocalin (NGAL) is a low molecular weight protein found in neutrophils, and plays a role in iron transport and sequestration.[125] In normal patients it can be found at low levels in both serum and urine. Because it may be elevated in the setting of inflammation, plasma NGAL is less specific than urinary NGAL in the detection of acute kidney injury.[131] Because NGAL is freely filtered by the glomerulus and fully reabsorbed, its presence in the urine is a marker of injury to the tubule or interstitium, making it a potentially useful clinical marker of renal injury. Both plasma and urinary NGAL levels have been shown to have excellent sensitivity and specificity in identifying acute kidney injury,[132] and the increase in NGAL occurs more than 24 hours before the increase in sCr. Aghel and colleagues[133] have shown that an elevated serum NGAL levels at the time of admission for ADHF is a strong predictor of WRF.

Kidney Injury Molecule 1

Kidney injury molecule 1 (KIM-1) is a transmembrane glycoprotein that is not found in the urine normally.[122] However, with acute tubular necrosis, the proximal tubule epithelial cells increase expression of KIM-1, and KIM-1 in the urine is associated with a 12-fold increased risk of acute tubular necrosis.[134] Of importance, the increase in KIM-1 levels occurs a full 24 hours before an increase in sCr.[135] There are minimal data on the use of KIM-1 in HF; however, Damman and colleagues[136] have shown that KIM-1 is elevated in stable HF patients with only mildly reduced GFR, suggesting ongoing tubular damage in these patients. These investigators also found that elevated levels were associated with an increased risk of death and hospitalization for HF, independent of GFR.[136]

N-Acetyl-β-ᴅ-Glucosaminidase

N-Acetyl-β-ᴅ-glucosaminidase (NAG) is a brush-border lysosomal enzyme that is shed from the proximal tubule cells in response to renal injury.[122,125] Its presence in the urine is an excellent predictor of acute kidney injury.[137–139] Similar to KIM-1, elevated NAG levels were found in HF patients with only mildly reduced GFR, and these elevations were associated with increased risk of death and hospitalization for HF, independent of GFR.[136]

Fatty Acid–Binding Protein

Fatty acid–binding proteins (FABPs) are proteins that bind selectively to free fatty acids and are expressed in a tissue-specific pattern.[122] FABP-1 and FABP-3 are found in the proximal and distal tubules, where they play a role in energy metabolism.[140] Their presence in urine is a sensitive and specific marker of acute kidney injury, and predicts the need for renal replacement therapy and death.[141] There are currently no data on the ability of FABP to predict WRF.

Albuminuria

Albumin is not filtered by the glomerulus under normal circumstances, and its presence in urine suggests a disruption of the basement membrane, which may be seen in a variety of diseases including diabetic and hypertensive kidney disease.[142,143] Albuminuria may be found in up to 32% of patients with HF,[144] and is thought to result from poor renal perfusion and increased congestion. Several studies have shown that the presence of albuminuria in HF is associated with increased mortality, even in the presence of normal GFR.[145,146]

SUMMARY

Renal dysfunction is a common, important comorbidity in patients with both chronic and acute HF. Both CKD and WRF are associated with worse outcomes, but our understanding of the complex bidirectional interactions between the heart and kidney remains poor. When addressing these interactions, one must consider the impact of intrinsic renal disease resulting from medical comorbidities on HF outcomes. In addition, WRF may result from any number of important processes, including RAAS and SNS activation, hemodynamics aberrations, pharmacotherapy, and inflammation. Understanding the role of each of these factors and their interplay is essential in fully understanding how to improve outcomes in patients with renal dysfunction and HF. It is hoped that the continued development of novel biomarkers of renal function will allow earlier diagnosis of WRF and ultimately allow earlier interventions that target renal protection.

REFERENCES

1. Effect of enalapril on survival in patients with reduced left ventricular ejection fractions and congestive heart failure. The SOLVD investigators. N Engl J Med 1991;325:293–302.

2. Effect of enalapril on mortality and the development of heart failure in asymptomatic patients with reduced left ventricular ejection fractions. The SOLVD investigators. N Engl J Med 1992;327:685–91.

3. Cleland JG, Carubelli V, Castiello T, et al. Renal dysfunction in acute and chronic heart failure: prevalence, incidence and prognosis. Heart Fail Rev 2012;17:133–49.

4. Dries DL, Exner DV, Domanski MJ, et al. The prognostic implications of renal insufficiency in asymptomatic and symptomatic patients with left ventricular systolic dysfunction. J Am Coll Cardiol 2000;35:681–9.

5. McMurray JJ, Ostergren J, Swedberg K, et al. Effects of candesartan in patients with chronic heart failure and reduced left-ventricular systolic function taking angiotensin-converting-enzyme inhibitors: the CHARM-ADDED trial. Lancet 2003;362:767–71.

6. Solomon SD, Wang D, Finn P, et al. Effect of candesartan on cause-specific mortality in heart failure patients: the Candesartan in Heart Failure Assessment of Reduction in Mortality and Morbidity (CHARM) program. Circulation 2004; 110:2180–3.

7. Yusuf S, Pfeffer MA, Swedberg K, et al. Effects of candesartan in patients with chronic heart failure and preserved left-ventricular ejection fraction: the CHARM-PRESERVED trial. Lancet 2003;362:777–81.

8. Zannad F, McMurray JJ, Krum H, et al. Eplerenone in patients with systolic heart failure and mild symptoms. N Engl J Med 2011;364:11–21.

9. de Silva R, Nikitin NP, Witte KK, et al. Incidence of renal dysfunction over 6 months in patients with chronic heart failure due to left ventricular systolic dysfunction: contributing factors and relationship to prognosis. Eur Heart J 2006;27:569–81.

10. Heywood JT, Fonarow GC, Costanzo MR, et al. High prevalence of renal dysfunction and its impact on outcome in 118,465 patients hospitalized with acute decompensated heart failure: a report from the ADHERE database. J Card Fail 2007;13:422–30.

11. Fonarow GC, Abraham WT, Albert NM, et al. Influence of a performance-improvement initiative on quality of care for patients hospitalized with heart failure: results of the Organized Program to Initiate Lifesaving Treatment in Hospitalized Patients with Heart Failure (OPTIMIZE-HF). Arch Intern Med 2007;167:1493–502.

12. Cleland JG, Swedberg K, Follath F, et al. The Euroheart Failure Survey Programme—a survey on the quality of care among patients with heart failure in Europe. Part 1: patient characteristics and diagnosis. Eur Heart J 2003;24: 442–63.

13. Cowie MR, Komajda M, Murray-Thomas T, et al. Prevalence and impact of worsening renal function in patients hospitalized with decompensated heart failure: results of the Prospective Outcomes study in Heart Failure (POSH). Eur Heart J 2006;27:1216–22.

14. Forman DE, Butler J, Wang Y, et al. Incidence, predictors at admission, and impact of worsening renal function among patients hospitalized with heart failure. J Am Coll Cardiol 2004;43:61–7.

15. Gottlieb SS, Abraham W, Butler J, et al. The prognostic importance of different definitions of worsening renal function in congestive heart failure. J Card Fail 2002;8:136–41.

16. Klein L, Massie BM, Leimberger JD, et al. Admission or changes in renal function during hospitalization for worsening heart failure predict postdischarge survival: results from the Outcomes of a Prospective Trial of Intravenous

Milrinone for Exacerbations of Chronic Heart Failure (OPTIME-CHF). Circ Heart Fail 2008;1:25–33.

17. Krumholz HM, Chen YT, Vaccarino V, et al. Correlates and impact on outcomes of worsening renal function in patients > or = 65 years of age with heart failure. Am J Cardiol 2000;85:1110–3.

18. Kociol RD, Greiner MA, Hammill BG, et al. Long-term outcomes of Medicare beneficiaries with worsening renal function during hospitalization for heart failure. Am J Cardiol 2010;105:1786–93.

19. Damman K, Navis G, Voors AA, et al. Worsening renal function and prognosis in heart failure: systematic review and meta-analysis. J Card Fail 2007;13: 599–608.

20. Ronco C, McCullough PA, Anker SD, et al. Cardiorenal syndromes: an executive summary from the consensus conference of the Acute Dialysis Quality Initiative (ADQI). Contrib Nephrol 2010;165:54–67.

21. Chittineni H, Miyawaki N, Gulipelli S, et al. Risk for acute renal failure in patients hospitalized for decompensated congestive heart failure. Am J Nephrol 2007; 27:55–62.

22. Giamouzis G, Butler J, Triposkiadis F. Renal function in advanced heart failure. Congest Heart Fail 2011;17:180–8.

23. Giamouzis G, Kalogeropoulos A, Georgiopoulou V, et al. Hospitalization epidemic in patients with heart failure: risk factors, risk prediction, knowledge gaps, and future directions. J Card Fail 2011;17:54–75.

24. Cruz DN, Gheorghiade M, Palazzuoli A, et al. Epidemiology and outcome of the cardio-renal syndrome. Heart Fail Rev 2011;16:531–42.

25. Smith GL, Lichtman JH, Bracken MB, et al. Renal impairment and outcomes in heart failure: systematic review and meta-analysis. J Am Coll Cardiol 2006;47: 1987–96.

26. McClellan WM, Flanders WD, Langston RD, et al. Anemia and renal insufficiency are independent risk factors for death among patients with congestive heart failure admitted to community hospitals: a population-based study. J Am Soc Nephrol 2002;13:1928–36.

27. McAlister FA, Ezekowitz J, Tonelli M, et al. Renal insufficiency and heart failure: prognostic and therapeutic implications from a prospective cohort study. Circulation 2004;109:1004–9.

28. National Kidney Foundation. K/DOQI clinical practice guidelines for chronic kidney disease: evaluation, classification, and stratification. Am J Kidney Dis 2002;39:S1–266.

29. Cockcroft DW, Gault MH. Prediction of creatinine clearance from serum creatinine. Nephron 1976;16:31–41.

30. Levey AS, Bosch JP, Lewis JB, et al. A more accurate method to estimate glomerular filtration rate from serum creatinine: a new prediction equation. Modification of diet in renal disease study group. Ann Intern Med 1999;130: 461–70.

31. Levey AS, Stevens LA, Schmid CH, et al. A new equation to estimate glomerular filtration rate. Ann Intern Med 2009;150:604–12.

32. Froissart M, Rossert J, Jacquot C, et al. Predictive performance of the modification of diet in renal disease and Cockcroft-Gault equations for estimating renal function. J Am Soc Nephrol 2005;16:763–73.

33. Smilde TD, van Veldhuisen DJ, Navis G, et al. Drawbacks and prognostic value of formulas estimating renal function in patients with chronic heart failure and systolic dysfunction. Circulation 2006;114:1572–80.

34. Zamora E, Lupon J, Vila J, et al. Estimated glomerular filtration rate and prognosis in heart failure: value of the Modification of Diet in Renal Disease Study-4, Chronic Kidney Disease Epidemiology Collaboration, and Cockcroft-Gault formulas. J Am Coll Cardiol 2012;59:1709–15.
35. Rich MW. Heart failure in the 21st century: a cardiogeriatric syndrome. J Gerontol A Biol Sci Med Sci 2001;56:M88–96.
36. Croft JB, Giles WH, Pollard RA, et al. Heart failure survival among older adults in the united states: a poor prognosis for an emerging epidemic in the Medicare population. Arch Intern Med 1999;159:505–10.
37. Lee DS, Gona P, Vasan RS, et al. Relation of disease pathogenesis and risk factors to heart failure with preserved or reduced ejection fraction: insights from the Framingham Heart Study of the National Heart, Lung, and Blood Institute. Circulation 2009;119:3070–7.
38. Lindeman RD, Tobin J, Shock NW. Longitudinal studies on the rate of decline in renal function with age. J Am Geriatr Soc 1985;33:278–85.
39. Perrone RD, Madias NE, Levey AS. Serum creatinine as an index of renal function: new insights into old concepts. Clin Chem 1992;38:1933–53.
40. Fehrman-Ekholm I, Skeppholm L. Renal function in the elderly (>70 years old) measured by means of iohexol clearance, serum creatinine, serum urea and estimated clearance. Scand J Urol Nephrol 2004;38:73–7.
41. Chrysochou C, Kalra PA. Current management of atherosclerotic renovascular disease—what have we learned from ASTRAL? Nephron Clin Pract 2010;115:c73–81.
42. van Ampting JM, Penne EL, Beek FJ, et al. Prevalence of atherosclerotic renal artery stenosis in patients starting dialysis. Nephrol Dial Transplant 2003;18:1147–51.
43. Mailloux LU, Napolitano B, Bellucci AG, et al. Renal vascular disease causing end-stage renal disease, incidence, clinical correlates, and outcomes: a 20-year clinical experience. Am J Kidney Dis 1994;24:622–9.
44. Olin JW, Melia M, Young JR, et al. Prevalence of atherosclerotic renal artery stenosis in patients with atherosclerosis elsewhere. Am J Med 1990;88:46N–51N.
45. Valle R, Aspromonte N, Carbonieri E, et al. Fall in readmission rate for heart failure after implementation of B-type natriuretic peptide testing for discharge decision: a retrospective study. Int J Cardiol 2008;126:400–6.
46. McClellan WM, Langston RD, Presley R. Medicare patients with cardiovascular disease have a high prevalence of chronic kidney disease and a high rate of progression to end-stage renal disease. J Am Soc Nephrol 2004;15:1912–9.
47. Philbin EF, DiSalvo TG. Prediction of hospital readmission for heart failure: development of a simple risk score based on administrative data. J Am Coll Cardiol 1999;33:1560–6.
48. Yamokoski LM, Hasselblad V, Moser DK, et al. Prediction of rehospitalization and death in severe heart failure by physicians and nurses of the ESCAPE trial. J Card Fail 2007;13:8–13.
49. Keenan PS, Normand SL, Lin Z, et al. An administrative claims measure suitable for profiling hospital performance on the basis of 30-day all-cause readmission rates among patients with heart failure. Circ Cardiovasc Qual Outcomes 2008;1:29–37.
50. Nohria A, Hasselblad V, Stebbins A, et al. Cardiorenal interactions: insights from the ESCAPE trial. J Am Coll Cardiol 2008;51:1268–74.
51. Doty JM, Saggi BH, Blocher CR, et al. Effects of increased renal parenchymal pressure on renal function. J Trauma 2000;48:874–7.
52. Malbrain ML, Deeren D, De Potter TJ. Intra-abdominal hypertension in the critically ill: it is time to pay attention. Curr Opin Crit Care 2005;11:156–71.

53. Butler J, Forman DE, Abraham WT, et al. Relationship between heart failure treatment and development of worsening renal function among hospitalized patients. Am Heart J 2004;147:331–8.

54. Packer M. The neurohormonal hypothesis: a theory to explain the mechanism of disease progression in heart failure. J Am Coll Cardiol 1992;20:248–54.

55. Packer M. Why do the kidneys release renin in patients with congestive heart failure? A nephrocentric view of converting-enzyme inhibition. Eur Heart J 1990;11(Suppl D): 44–52.

56. Brecher P. Angiotensin II and cardiac fibrosis. Trends Cardiovasc Med 1996;6: 193–8.

57. Brilla CG, Pick R, Tan LB, et al. Remodeling of the rat right and left ventricles in experimental hypertension. Circ Res 1990;67:1355–64.

58. McEwan PE, Gray GA, Sherry L, et al. Differential effects of angiotensin ii on cardiac cell proliferation and intramyocardial perivascular fibrosis in vivo. Circulation 1998;98:2765–73.

59. Lijnen P, Petrov V. Induction of cardiac fibrosis by aldosterone. J Mol Cell Cardiol 2000;32:865–79.

60. Lijnen PJ, Petrov VV, Fagard RH. Induction of cardiac fibrosis by angiotensin II. Methods Find Exp Clin Pharmacol 2000;22:709–23.

61. Mezzano SA, Ruiz-Ortega M, Egido J. Angiotensin II and renal fibrosis. Hypertension 2001;38:635–8.

62. Ruiz-Ortega M, Gonzalez S, Seron D, et al. ACE inhibition reduces proteinuria, glomerular lesions and extracellular matrix production in a normotensive rat model of immune complex nephritis. Kidney Int 1995;48:1778–91.

63. Ruiz-Ortega M, Lorenzo O, Suzuki Y, et al. Proinflammatory actions of angiotensins. Curr Opin Nephrol Hypertens 2001;10:321–9.

64. Ruiz-Ortega M, Lorenzo O, Ruperez M, et al. Systemic infusion of angiotensin ii into normal rats activates nuclear factor-kappaB and AP-1 in the kidney: role of AT(1) and AT(2) receptors. Am J Pathol 2001;158:1743–56.

65. Converse RL Jr, Jacobsen TN, Toto RD, et al. Sympathetic overactivity in patients with chronic renal failure. N Engl J Med 1992;327:1912–8.

66. Zoccali C, Mallamaci F, Parlongo S, et al. Plasma norepinephrine predicts survival and incident cardiovascular events in patients with end-stage renal disease. Circulation 2002;105:1354–9.

67. DiBona GF. Nervous kidney. Interaction between renal sympathetic nerves and the renin-angiotensin system in the control of renal function. Hypertension 2000; 36:1083–8.

68. Salomonsson M, Brannstrom K, Arendshorst WJ. Alpha(1)-adrenoceptor subtypes in rat renal resistance vessels: in vivo and in vitro studies. Am J Physiol Renal Physiol 2000;278:F138–47.

69. Bakris GL, Hart P, Ritz E. Beta blockers in the management of chronic kidney disease. Kidney Int 2006;70:1905–13.

70. Osborn JL, DiBona GF, Thames MD. Beta-1 receptor mediation of renin secretion elicited by low-frequency renal nerve stimulation. J Pharmacol Exp Ther 1981;216:265–9.

71. Jovanovic D, Jovovic D, Mihailovic-Stanojevic N, et al. Influence of carvedilol on chronic renal failure progression in spontaneously hypertensive rats with adriamycin nephropathy. Clin Nephrol 2005;63:446–53.

72. Akhter MW, Aronson D, Bitar F, et al. Effect of elevated admission serum creatinine and its worsening on outcome in hospitalized patients with decompensated heart failure. Am J Cardiol 2004;94:957–60.

73. Hillege HL, Girbes AR, de Kam PJ, et al. Renal function, neurohormonal activation, and survival in patients with chronic heart failure. Circulation 2000;102: 203–10.
74. Hillege HL, Nitsch D, Pfeffer MA, et al. Renal function as a predictor of outcome in a broad spectrum of patients with heart failure. Circulation 2006;113:671–8.
75. Ljungman S, Laragh JH, Cody RJ. Role of the kidney in congestive heart failure. Relationship of cardiac index to kidney function. Drugs 1990;39(Suppl 4):10–21 [discussion: 22–4].
76. Mullens W, Abrahams Z, Skouri HN, et al. Elevated intra-abdominal pressure in acute decompensated heart failure: a potential contributor to worsening renal function? J Am Coll Cardiol 2008;51:300–6.
77. Damman K, van Deursen VM, Navis G, et al. Increased central venous pressure is associated with impaired renal function and mortality in a broad spectrum of patients with cardiovascular disease. J Am Coll Cardiol 2009;53:582–8.
78. Mullens W, Abrahams Z, Francis GS, et al. Importance of venous congestion for worsening of renal function in advanced decompensated heart failure. J Am Coll Cardiol 2009;53:589–96.
79. Guglin M, Rivero A, Matar F, et al. Renal dysfunction in heart failure is due to congestion but not low output. Clin Cardiol 2011;34:113–6.
80. Testani JM, McCauley BD, Kimmel SE, et al. Characteristics of patients with improvement or worsening in renal function during treatment of acute decompensated heart failure. Am J Cardiol 2010;106:1763–9.
81. Adams KF Jr, Fonarow GC, Emerman CL, et al. Characteristics and outcomes of patients hospitalized for heart failure in the United States: rationale, design, and preliminary observations from the first 100,000 cases in the Acute Decompensated Heart Failure National Registry (ADHERE). Am Heart J 2005;149:209–16.
82. Cooper HA, Dries DL, Davis CE, et al. Diuretics and risk of arrhythmic death in patients with left ventricular dysfunction. Circulation 1999;100:1311–5.
83. Ahmed A, Husain A, Love TE, et al. Heart failure, chronic diuretic use, and increase in mortality and hospitalization: an observational study using propensity score methods. Eur Heart J 2006;27:1431–9.
84. Eshaghian S, Horwich TB, Fonarow GC. Relation of loop diuretic dose to mortality in advanced heart failure. Am J Cardiol 2006;97:1759–64.
85. Domanski M, Norman J, Pitt B, et al. Diuretic use, progressive heart failure, and death in patients in the Studies of Left Ventricular Dysfunction (SOLVD). J Am Coll Cardiol 2003;42:705–8.
86. Francis GS, Benedict C, Johnstone DE, et al. Comparison of neuroendocrine activation in patients with left ventricular dysfunction with and without congestive heart failure. A substudy of the Studies of Left Ventricular Dysfunction (SOLVD). Circulation 1990;82:1724–9.
87. Metra M, Nodari S, Parrinello G, et al. Worsening renal function in patients hospitalised for acute heart failure: clinical implications and prognostic significance. Eur J Heart Fail 2008;10:188–95.
88. Hasselblad V, Gattis Stough W, Shah MR, et al. Relation between dose of loop diuretics and outcomes in a heart failure population: results of the escape trial. Eur J Heart Fail 2007;9:1064–9.
89. Carubelli V, Metra M, Lombardi C, et al. Renal dysfunction in acute heart failure: epidemiology, mechanisms and assessment. Heart Fail Rev 2012;17:271–82.
90. Testani JM, Chen J, McCauley BD, et al. Potential effects of aggressive decongestion during the treatment of decompensated heart failure on renal function and survival. Circulation 2010;122:265–72.

91. Felker GM, Lee KL, Bull DA, et al. Diuretic strategies in patients with acute decompensated heart failure. N Engl J Med 2011;364:797–805.

92. Effects of enalapril on mortality in severe congestive heart failure. Results of the Cooperative North Scandinavian Enalapril Survival Study (CONSENSUS). The CONSENSUS Trial Study Group. N Engl J Med 1987;316:1429–35.

93. Bakris GL, Weir MR. Angiotensin-converting enzyme inhibitor-associated elevations in serum creatinine: is this a cause for concern? Arch Intern Med 2000;160: 685–93.

94. Ruiz-Ortega M, Ruperez M, Lorenzo O, et al. Angiotensin II regulates the synthesis of proinflammatory cytokines and chemokines in the kidney. Kidney Int Suppl 2002;82:S12–22.

95. Ljungman S, Kjekshus J, Swedberg K. Renal function in severe congestive heart failure during treatment with enalapril (the Cooperative North Scandinavian Enalapril Survival Study [CONSENSUS] trial). Am J Cardiol 1992;70:479–87.

96. Oster JR, Materson BJ. Renal and electrolyte complications of congestive heart failure and effects of therapy with angiotensin-converting enzyme inhibitors. Arch Intern Med 1992;152:704–10.

97. Valika AA, Gheorghiade M. Ace inhibitor therapy for heart failure in patients with impaired renal function: a review of the literature. Heart Fail Rev 2012. [Epub ahead of print].

98. Colombo PC, Ganda A, Lin J, et al. Inflammatory activation: cardiac, renal, and cardio-renal interactions in patients with the cardiorenal syndrome. Heart Fail Rev 2012;17:177–90.

99. Ferrari R, Bachetti T, Confortini R, et al. Tumor necrosis factor soluble receptors in patients with various degrees of congestive heart failure. Circulation 1995;92: 1479–86.

100. Testa M, Yeh M, Lee P, et al. Circulating levels of cytokines and their endogenous modulators in patients with mild to severe congestive heart failure due to coronary artery disease or hypertension. J Am Coll Cardiol 1996;28:964–71.

101. Maeda K, Tsutamoto T, Wada A, et al. High levels of plasma brain natriuretic peptide and interleukin-6 after optimized treatment for heart failure are independent risk factors for morbidity and mortality in patients with congestive heart failure. J Am Coll Cardiol 2000;36:1587–93.

102. Kozdag G, Ertas G, Kilic T, et al. Elevated level of high-sensitivity C-reactive protein is important in determining prognosis in chronic heart failure. Med Sci Monit 2010;16:CR156–61.

103. Alonso-Martinez JL, Llorente-Diez B, Echegaray-Agara M, et al. C-reactive protein as a predictor of improvement and readmission in heart failure. Eur J Heart Fail 2002;4:331–6.

104. Kalra D, Sivasubramanian N, Mann DL. Angiotensin ii induces tumor necrosis factor biosynthesis in the adult mammalian heart through a protein kinase C-dependent pathway. Circulation 2002;105:2198–205.

105. Moriyama T, Fujibayashi M, Fujiwara Y, et al. Angiotensin II stimulates interleukin-6 release from cultured mouse mesangial cells. J Am Soc Nephrol 1995;6:95–101.

106. Murray DR, Prabhu SD, Chandrasekar B. Chronic beta-adrenergic stimulation induces myocardial proinflammatory cytokine expression. Circulation 2000; 101:2338–41.

107. Prabhu SD, Chandrasekar B, Murray DR, et al. Beta-adrenergic blockade in developing heart failure: effects on myocardial inflammatory cytokines, nitric oxide, and remodeling. Circulation 2000;101:2103–9.

108. Colombo PC, Banchs JE, Celaj S, et al. Endothelial cell activation in patients with decompensated heart failure. Circulation 2005;111:58–62.

109. Colombo PC, Rastogi S, Onat D, et al. Activation of endothelial cells in conduit veins of dogs with heart failure and veins of normal dogs after vascular stretch by acute volume loading. J Card Fail 2009;15:457–63.

110. Anker SD, Egerer KR, Volk HD, et al. Elevated soluble CD14 receptors and altered cytokines in chronic heart failure. Am J Cardiol 1997;79:1426–30.

111. Niebauer J, Volk HD, Kemp M, et al. Endotoxin and immune activation in chronic heart failure: a prospective cohort study. Lancet 1999;353:1838–42.

112. Peschel T, Schonauer M, Thiele H, et al. Invasive assessment of bacterial endotoxin and inflammatory cytokines in patients with acute heart failure. Eur J Heart Fail 2003;5:609–14.

113. Yhee JY, Yu CH, Kim JH, et al. Effects of T lymphocytes, interleukin-1, and interleukin-6 on renal fibrosis in canine end-stage renal disease. J Vet Diagn Invest 2008;20:585–92.

114. Szeto CC, Kwan BC, Chow KM, et al. Endotoxemia is related to systemic inflammation and atherosclerosis in peritoneal dialysis patients. Clin J Am Soc Nephrol 2008;3:431–6.

115. Schwedler SB, Guderian F, Dammrich J, et al. Tubular staining of modified C-reactive protein in diabetic chronic kidney disease. Nephrol Dial Transplant 2003;18:2300–7.

116. Radeke HH, Meier B, Topley N, et al. Interleukin 1-alpha and tumor necrosis factor-alpha induce oxygen radical production in mesangial cells. Kidney Int 1990;37:767–75.

117. DiPetrillo K, Coutermarsh B, Gesek FA. Urinary tumor necrosis factor contributes to sodium retention and renal hypertrophy during diabetes. Am J Physiol Renal Physiol 2003;284:F113–21.

118. Garvin JL, Ortiz PA. The role of reactive oxygen species in the regulation of tubular function. Acta Physiol Scand 2003;179:225–32.

119. Taddei S, Favilla S, Duranti P, et al. Vascular renin-angiotensin system and neurotransmission in hypertensive persons. Hypertension 1991;18:266–77.

120. Fiksen-Olsen MJ, Strick DM, Hawley H, et al. Renal effects of angiotensin II inhibition during increases in renal venous pressure. Hypertension 1992;19:II137–41.

121. Kastner PR, Hall JE, Guyton AC. Renal hemodynamic responses to increased renal venous pressure: role of angiotensin II. Am J Physiol 1982;243:F260–4.

122. Damman K, Voors AA, Navis G, et al. Current and novel renal biomarkers in heart failure. Heart Fail Rev 2012;17:241–50.

123. Fonarow GC, Adams KF Jr, Abraham WT, et al. Risk stratification for in-hospital mortality in acutely decompensated heart failure: classification and regression tree analysis. JAMA 2005;293:572–80.

124. Aronson D, Mittleman MA, Burger AJ. Elevated blood urea nitrogen level as a predictor of mortality in patients admitted for decompensated heart failure. Am J Med 2004;116:466–73.

125. Comnick M, Ishani A. Renal biomarkers of kidney injury in cardiorenal syndrome. Curr Heart Fail Rep 2011;8:99–105.

126. Laterza OF, Price CP, Scott MG. Cystatin C: an improved estimator of glomerular filtration rate? Clin Chem 2002;48:699–707.

127. Newman DJ, Thakkar H, Edwards RG, et al. Serum cystatin C measured by automated immunoassay: a more sensitive marker of changes in GFR than serum creatinine. Kidney Int 1995;47:312–8.

128. Hoek FJ, Kemperman FA, Krediet RT. A comparison between cystatin C, plasma creatinine and the Cockcroft and Gault formula for the estimation of glomerular filtration rate. Nephrol Dial Transplant 2003;18:2024–31.

129. Tidman M, Sjostrom P, Jones I. A comparison of GFR estimating formulae based upon S-cystatin C and S-creatinine and a combination of the two. Nephrol Dial Transplant 2008;23:154–60.

130. Lassus J, Harjola VP, Sund R, et al. Prognostic value of cystatin C in acute heart failure in relation to other markers of renal function and NT-proBNP. Eur Heart J 2007;28:1841–7.

131. Schmidt-Ott KM, Mori K, Li JY, et al. Dual action of neutrophil gelatinase-associated lipocalin. J Am Soc Nephrol 2007;18:407–13.

132. Mishra J, Dent C, Tarabishi R, et al. Neutrophil gelatinase-associated lipocalin (NGAL) as a biomarker for acute renal injury after cardiac surgery. Lancet 2005;365:1231–8.

133. Aghel A, Shrestha K, Mullens W, et al. Serum neutrophil gelatinase-associated lipocalin (NGAL) in predicting worsening renal function in acute decompensated heart failure. J Card Fail 2010;16:49–54.

134. Han WK, Bailly V, Abichandani R, et al. Kidney injury molecule-1 (KIM-1): a novel biomarker for human renal proximal tubule injury. Kidney Int 2002;62:237–44.

135. Han WK, Waikar SS, Johnson A, et al. Urinary biomarkers in the early diagnosis of acute kidney injury. Kidney Int 2008;73:863–9.

136. Damman K, Van Veldhuisen DJ, Navis G, et al. Tubular damage in chronic systolic heart failure is associated with reduced survival independent of glomerular filtration rate. Heart 2010;96:1297–302.

137. Westhuyzen J, Endre ZH, Reece G, et al. Measurement of tubular enzymuria facilitates early detection of acute renal impairment in the intensive care unit. Nephrol Dial Transplant 2003;18:543–51.

138. Bazzi C, Petrini C, Rizza V, et al. Urinary N-acetyl-beta-glucosaminidase excretion is a marker of tubular cell dysfunction and a predictor of outcome in primary glomerulonephritis. Nephrol Dial Transplant 2002;17:1890–6.

139. Liangos O, Perianayagam MC, Vaidya VS, et al. Urinary N-acetyl-beta-(D)-glucosaminidase activity and kidney injury molecule-1 level are associated with adverse outcomes in acute renal failure. J Am Soc Nephrol 2007;18:904–12.

140. Maatman RG, Van Kuppevelt TH, Veerkamp JH. Two types of fatty acid-binding protein in human kidney. Isolation, characterization and localization. Biochem J 1991;273(Pt 3):759–66.

141. Ferguson MA, Vaidya VS, Waikar SS, et al. Urinary liver-type fatty acid-binding protein predicts adverse outcomes in acute kidney injury. Kidney Int 2010;77:708–14.

142. Agewall S, Wikstrand J, Ljungman S, et al. Usefulness of microalbuminuria in predicting cardiovascular mortality in treated hypertensive men with and without diabetes mellitus. Risk Factor Intervention Study Group. Am J Cardiol 1997;80:164–9.

143. Mogensen CE. Microalbuminuria predicts clinical proteinuria and early mortality in maturity-onset diabetes. N Engl J Med 1984;310:356–60.

144. van de Wal RM, Asselbergs FW, Plokker HW, et al. High prevalence of microalbuminuria in chronic heart failure patients. J Card Fail 2005;11:602–6.

145. Jackson CE, Solomon SD, Gerstein HC, et al. Albuminuria in chronic heart failure: prevalence and prognostic importance. Lancet 2009;374:543–50.

146. Masson S, Latini R, Milani V, et al. Prevalence and prognostic value of elevated urinary albumin excretion in patients with chronic heart failure: data from the GISSI-heart failure trial. Circ Heart Fail 2010;3:65–72.

Management of Comorbid Conditions in Heart Failure
A Review

Vijaiganesh Nagarajan, MD, MRCP[a], W.H. Wilson Tang, MD[b],*

KEYWORDS

- Heart failure • Co-morbid conditions

KEY POINTS

- Diabetes mellitus can affect cardiac function at the cellular level through different mechanisms such as myocyte fibrosis, intramyocardial microangiopathy, and cardiac autonomic imbalance, causing diabetic cardiomyopathy.
- Angiotensin-converting enzyme inhibitors have been proved to have mortality benefit in patients with systolic heart failure irrespective of the diabetic status.
- Recent practice guidelines[1] recommend angiotensin-converting enzyme inhibitors and β-blockers as first-line therapy for asymptomatic hypertensive patients with demonstrable left ventricular dysfunction.

INTRODUCTION

Heart failure is a chronic and progressive condition, and is a major cause of morbidity and mortality worldwide. More than 5.8 million people in United States have a diagnosis of heart failure, and the estimated annual cost of heart failure is around US$37.2 billion.[2] Recent insights have emerged to show that heart failure is a complex clinical condition, particularly in the elderly, that usually interacts with other chronic medical conditions via known and possibly yet unknown mechanisms. This review discusses the common comorbid conditions, their interactions with heart failure, and treatment options. Several major comorbidities that are important in management of heart failure, such as cardiorenal syndrome, atrial fibrillation, and malignancy, are discussed in reviews elsewhere in this issue and are therefore not discussed here.

EPIDEMIOLOGY OF COMORBID CONDITIONS IN HEART FAILURE

The prevalence of comorbid conditions in heart failure varies depending on study population and severity of heart failure. It may also vary secondary to different definitions

[a] Department of Hospital Medicine, Cleveland Clinic, Cleveland OH, USA; [b] Heart and Vascular Institute, Cleveland Clinic, Cleveland OH, USA
* Corresponding author.
E-mail address: tangw@ccf.org

Med Clin N Am 96 (2012) 975–985
http://dx.doi.org/10.1016/j.mcna.2012.07.006
0025-7125/12/$ – see front matter © 2012 Elsevier Inc. All rights reserved.

medical.theclinics.com

used in different studies. In a large cross-sectional study involving 122,630 US Medicare beneficiaries who have heart failure and are 65 years or older, Braunstein and colleagues[3] examined the relationship of 20 most common noncardiac comorbidities to potentially preventable hospitalizations and total mortality at 1 year. Forty percent of patients in this sample had 5 or more predefined comorbidities. Also, the risk of hospitalization significantly increased with the number of chronic conditions. The 5 common comorbid conditions in this study, in decreasing prevalence, were hypertension (55%), diabetes mellitus (31%), chronic obstructive pulmonary disease (COPD)/bronchiectasis (26%), ocular disorders (24%), and hypercholesterolemia (21%). Another interesting study evaluated 1395 patients with self-reported heart failure using the National Health and Nutrition Examination Survey (NHANES) database.[4] The proportion of heart failure patients with 5 or more comorbidities increased from 42% to 58% during the past 2 decades. The main comorbid conditions responsible for this increase were hypercholesterolemia, diabetes, obesity, and kidney disease. Although this could represent increasing prevalence of these comorbid conditions during the study period, there has also been better screening for comorbid conditions and recognition of obesity as a chronic health problem in recent years. Wong and colleagues[4] examined the trend in medications during the same period (1988–2008). Although the use of digoxin and calcium-channel blockers decreased over time, they noted that the prescription drug use increased from a mean of 4.1 to 6.4 prescription medications. A separate cost analysis of comorbid conditions investigated 1266 Medicare beneficiaries with heart failure, and demonstrated that the presence of comorbid conditions significantly increased the Medicare expenditure.[5] Furthermore, 81% of patients had at least 1 predefined comorbid condition, and the noncardiac comorbidities that were associated with increased mean expenditure included hemiplegia/paraplegia, renal disease, peripheral vascular disease, and dementia.

DIABETES MELLITUS

Diabetes mellitus is an independent risk factor for the development of heart failure, which was clearly demonstrated in the Framingham Heart Study involving 5209 subjects.[6] Study investigators noted a 2-fold increase in incidence of heart failure in men and a greater than 5-fold increase in women during a 20-year surveillance. A large, prospective, observational trial from the United Kingdom (UK Prospective Diabetes Study) involving 3642 patients showed that the risk of heart failure decreased by 16% per 1% reduction in hemoglobin A1c.[7] There was also a 14% reduction in myocardial infarction for every 1% reduction in hemoglobin A1c, which is another important predictor of future risk of heart failure. Diabetes also proved to be an independent predictor of mortality in patients with heart failure. The DIAMOND (Danish Investigations and Arrhythmia ON Dofetilide) study investigators[8] evaluated 5491 patients who were hospitalized with heart failure, and identified relative risk of death in diabetic patients in this study as being 1.5 (95% confidence interval [CI], 1.3–1.6, $P<.0001$), even after adjusting for hypertension, ischemic heart disease, and other risk factors. Similar results were shown in the Studies of Left Ventricular Dysfunction (SOLVD) trial in patients with ischemic cardiomyopathy.[9]

Although there is clear evidence of increased risk and poor prognosis with diabetes mellitus, the pathophysiologic mechanism is less clear. Diabetes mellitus can affect cardiac function at the cellular level through differing mechanisms such as myocyte fibrosis, intramyocardial microangiopathy, and cardiac autonomic imbalance, causing diabetic cardiomyopathy.[10] Diabetic cardiomyopathy, along with coexistent myocardial ischemia and hypertension/ventricular hypertrophy, is referred to as the cardiotoxic triad, which attempts to explain the common mechanisms of poor cardiac function in patients with diabetes mellitus.[11] The choice of glucose-lowering medications may be controversial in patients with heart failure. Although metformin has traditionally been linked to lactic acidosis in heart failure, it was the only antidiabetic agent that was associated with decreased all-cause mortality in a contemporary systematic review.[12] By contrast, thiazolidinedione use has been linked to an increased risk of fluid retention[13] and hence is not used commonly in patients with advanced heart failure.

Angiotensin-converting enzyme (ACE) inhibitors have been proved to have mortality benefit in patients with systolic heart failure, regardless of the diabetic status, in a subgroup analysis of meta-analysis of major clinical trials,[14] which compared 2398 patients with diabetes and 10,188 patients without diabetes. The relative risk (RR) of mortality due to ACE inhibitors was similar in diabetic and nondiabetic patients (RR of 0.84 vs 0.85). The same meta-analysis also evaluated efficacy of β-blockers in patients with and without diabetes. Although β-blockers showed mortality benefit in both groups, relative reduction in mortality was less for diabetic patients (RR of 0.77 vs 0.65), but there was no statistical significance. The historic concern of hypoglycemic unawareness with β-blockers is not well proved[15] and definitely does not outweigh the benefits of β-blockers. The mortality benefit of aldosterone antagonists was similar in patients with and without diabetes.[16]

HYPERTENSION

Hypertension is one of the two major causes of heart failure.[17] The other cause, coronary artery disease, most often coexists with or is secondary to hypertension, making hypertension the most common risk factor for heart failure. Data suggest that up to 75% of patients with heart failure may have antecedent hypertension.[2] Hypertension as a risk factor for heart failure was demonstrated in a large study that included 5143 subjects aged 40 to 89 years and a mean follow-up of longer than 14 years.[18] Subjects with hypertension had a 2- to 3-fold increased risk of developing heart failure compared with normotensive subjects. Of the major risk factors examined in this study, hypertension had the highest prevalence (60%), but myocardial infarction had the highest hazard ratio for developing heart failure. There are multiple studies, starting from the early years of heart failure investigation, that support the fact that appropriate treatment of hypertension can dramatically decrease the risk of developing heart failure. This was well demonstrated in the Systolic Hypertension in Elderly (SHEP) trial, which randomized 4736 patients to active treatment of hypertension versus placebo.[19] The incidence of left ventricular failure was 50% lower in the treatment group (RR, 0.46; 95% CI, 0.33–0.65). Decreased incidence of myocardial infarction was also noted in the treatment group of this study. Similar results were noted in patients older than 70 years.[20]

Hypertension is the most common cause of left ventricular hypertrophy, which is a strong predictor of adverse cardiac events including heart failure.[21] Pressure overload from systolic hypertension causes myocardial architectural changes such as myocardial hypertrophy and fibrosis.[22] Thereby, hypertension remains an important cause of diastolic dysfunction, which is a contributory factor in a major proportion of patients with heart failure. Diastolic dysfunction could precede systolic dysfunction in hypertensive heart failure.[23] The choice of antihypertensive medications in patients with heart failure is relatively easy, as most of the medications used for the treatment of heart failure also control blood pressure. Recent practice guidelines[1] recommend ACE inhibitors and β-blockers as first-line therapy for asymptomatic hypertensive patients with demonstrable left ventricular dysfunction. In addition, the guidelines also recommend angiotensin II receptor blockers, aldosterone receptor antagonists, and loop diuretics in patients with symptoms.

HYPERLIPIDEMIA

Advanced heart failure is commonly perceived as a cachectic disease. However, a history of hyperlipidemia is among the top 5 comorbid conditions in patients with heart failure. Hyperlipidemia is not a predictor of poor prognosis in patients with heart failure, and elevated cholesterol levels were paradoxically associated with a better survival rate. This phenomenon is called reverse epidemiology.[24] Meanwhile, the use of statin therapy in patients with heart failure has been explored. The Controlled Rosuvastatin Multinational Study in Heart Failure (CORONA) trial[25] randomized 5011 elderly patients with ischemic cardiomyopathy to rosuvastatin and placebo. Despite the reduction in low-density lipoprotein and high-sensitivity C-reactive protein levels, there was no significant difference in the primary end point, but there were fewer hospitalizations for cardiovascular causes in the rosuvastatin group. By contrast, in the Gruppo Italiano per lo Studio della Sopravvivenza nell'Infarto Miocardico–Heart Failure (GISSI-HF) trial,[26] 4574 adult patients with heart failure were randomized, but the trial also included patients with nonischemic cardiomyopathy and heart failure with preserved ejection fraction. There was no difference in either primary or secondary end points, including hospitalizations for cardiac reasons.

Coenzyme Q10 (CoQ10) plays an important role in the synthesis of mitochondrial adenosine triphosphate. Low levels of CoQ10 have been shown to be an independent predictor of mortality in patients with heart failure.[27] Because statins are known to decrease CoQ10 levels, there was a concern regarding the use of statins in patients with heart failure, which was addressed in a substudy of the CORONA trial.[28] Although rosuvastatin decreased CoQ10 levels, rosuvastatin treatment was not associated with worse outcomes. Meanwhile, CoQ10 supplementation itself has yet to demonstrate significant long-term benefits. Further randomized controlled trials may be needed to clarify the role of statins and CoQ10 supplementation in patients with heart failure.

CHRONIC OBSTRUCTIVE PULMONARY DISEASE

COPD is a frequent comorbidity in patients with heart failure, with prevalence ranging from 20% to 30%. COPD and heart failure share common risk factors such as smoking and age. Smoking causes local airway inflammation leading to airway obstruction, but at same time can cause systemic inflammation and endothelial dysfunction. Another hypothesis is that COPD itself causes low-grade systemic inflammation[29] and hence may play an important role in the progression of cardiovascular disease. Because the clinical presentations of these conditions can be similar, there may be a delay in diagnosing the concomitant disease condition. Misdiagnosis or delay in the diagnosis of heart failure causes morbidity and an increase in treatment cost,[30] and vice versa. Although clinical examination will provide clues, plasma B-type natriuretic peptide is increasingly used to differentiate both conditions.[31] It is noteworthy that "cardiogenic wheezing" is also common in advanced heart failure.

COPD was found to be an independent predictor of mortality in patients with heart failure in multiple studies.[32] Forced expiratory volume in 1 second (FEV$_1$) was found to be as important as cholesterol in predicting cardiovascular mortality.[33] Smoking cessation is the mainstay of treatment for COPD, which decreases the incidence of cardiovascular diseases as well.[34] A meta-analysis showed that β-adrenergic agonists that are commonly used to treat COPD significantly increased the risk of cardiovascular events such as tachycardia, atrial fibrillation, myocardial infarction, and heart failure.[35]

Many physicians perceive COPD as a contraindication to β-blockers. However, a Cochrane review of 22 studies evaluating adverse effects of cardioselective β-blockers in patients with COPD found no significant change in FEV_1 or respiratory symptoms. Subgroup analysis was done for severe COPD and reversible airway obstruction, and the results were unchanged.[36] Hence, cardioselective β-blockers can be safely prescribed to patients with both COPD and heart failure.

SLEEP-DISORDERED BREATHING

Sleep-disordered breathing (SDB) is recently gaining recognition in the heart failure literature. The 2 forms of SDB are obstructive sleep apnea (OSA) and central sleep apnea (CSA). The incidence of sleep apnea is likely to increase because of increasing obesity and aging of the general population, while there has been a long-standing association between advanced heart failure and CSA ("Cheyne-Stokes breathing"). There are multiple mechanisms through which OSA may affect the cardiovascular system: intermittent hypoxia, systemic inflammation, negative intrathoracic pressure, and elevated blood pressure.[37] OSA was associated with an increased risk of atrial fibrillation,[38] which itself has a deleterious effect on cardiac function in patients with heart failure. In an observational study involving 4422 patients with OSA, OSA emerged as an independent predictor of coronary artery disease and heart failure in men. In this study, men with an apnea-hypopnea index (AHI: average number of apneas plus hypopneas per hour of sleep) of 30 or higher were 58% more likely to develop heart failure in comparison with those with an AHI of less than 5.[39] A prospective trial from Canada followed 164 systolic patients with heart failure for 2.9 years.[40] In this trial, untreated OSA (AHI ≥15) was independently associated with increased mortality risk compared with patients with mild or no OSA.

In patients with undiagnosed SDB, a high index of suspicion is necessary to screen and diagnose SDB. In a recent retrospective study involving 30,719 Medicare beneficiaries, 1263 patients were clinically suspected to have OSA.[41] Patients who were tested and treated for OSA had a better 2-year prognosis than patients who did not undergo testing (hazard ratio, 0.33; 95% CI, 0.21–0.51; $P<.0001$). Also, of the patients who underwent testing, treated patients had a better 2-year survival rate compared with those who were untreated. The Canadian Continuous Positive Airway Pressure for Patients with Central Sleep Apnea and Heart Failure (CANPAP) study randomly assigned 258 patients with heart failure and CSA to receive continuous positive airway pressure (CPAP) or no CPAP. CPAP improved nocturnal oxygenation, left ventricular ejection fraction, and 6-minute walk distance, but failed to improve survival.[42] The reason for this finding was unclear at the time, but a post hoc analysis published couple of years later showed that mortality benefit was observed in patients whose CSA was well suppressed with CPAP, with no benefit for those patients whose CSA was unsuppressed.[43]

ANEMIA

The prognostic significance of anemia in multiple other disease states is well established. Prevalence varies widely among studies depending on the definition of anemia and the severity of underlying heart failure. Groenveld and colleagues[44] examined the role of anemia in a large meta-analysis involving 153,180 patients with heart failure; 37.2% of the patients were anemic and crude mortality was significantly higher in anemic patients (odds ratio, 1.96; 95% CI, 1.72–2.21). This difference was noted in both diastolic and systolic heart failure and persisted even after adjustment for known confounders. The cause of anemia is multifactorial, although functional iron deficiency has been a strong postulate. Chronic inflammation, hemodilution, bone marrow dysfunction, renal dysfunction, and hematinic deficiencies are some mechanisms worthy of note.[45] The renin-angiotensin system plays a role in erythropoiesis, hence ACE inhibitors or angiotensin II receptor blockers may be associated with decreased erythropoietin levels. On the other hand, blood transfusions have been shown to be associated with higher mortality in the setting of acute coronary syndromes, hence blood transfusions are falling out of favor in heart failure also. There is no clear hemoglobin cutoff below which transfusion may be recommended in patients with heart failure.

The interest is diverted toward 2 other possible modes of treatment: intravenous iron and erythropoietin-stimulating agents. A prospective observational study involving 546 stable patients with systolic heart failure found that 57% of anemic patients are iron deficient based on iron studies.[46] Of interest, they also noted that about 32% of patients without anemia also had iron deficiency. Iron-deficiency anemia was an independent predictor of mortality or need for transplantation in this study. The treatment aspect of iron deficiency was examined in the Ferric carboxymaltose Assessment in patients with IRon deficiency and chronic Heart Failure with and without anemia (FAIR-HF) trial,[47] which enrolled 459 patients with systolic dysfunction and iron deficiency. Treatment with intravenous iron improved symptoms, functional capacity, and quality of life, but there was no difference in mortality, and results were the same regardless of the presence of anemia. Meanwhile, the Study of Anemia in Heart Failure Trial (STAMINA-HeFT) randomized 319 patients with systolic heart failure with moderate anemia to receive darbepoetin or placebo. Patients in the darbepoetin arm did not demonstrate significant improvement in exercise duration or quality of life, but there was a trend toward lower all-cause mortality or first heart failure hospitalization.[48] With concerns raised by recent clinical trials on the use of these erythropoietin-stimulating agents,[49] large prospective heart failure clinical trials are ongoing to clarify their potential utility.

OBESITY

Increasing body mass index (BMI) increases the risk of developing heart failure, which could be due to coexisting cardiovascular risk factors in obese subjects. However, BMI is also known to be an independent risk factor for heart failure. This was demonstrated in 5881 patients from the Framingham Heart Study, in whom there was a 5% to 7% increase in risk of heart failure for every unit increase in BMI.[50] In fact, obesity-related cardiomyopathy (adipositas cordis) was described as early as 1818 by Cheyne.[51] There are multiple mechanisms through which obesity can cause heart failure, including left ventricular hypertrophy, diastolic dysfunction, and systolic dysfunction. Although obesity increases the risk of developing heart failure, the same is not true when it comes to prognosis. At the other end of the spectrum, obesity improves the prognosis of patients with advanced heart failure ("obesity paradox"), as demonstrated in a meta-analysis that included 28,209 patients with heart failure.[52] Overweight and obesity were associated with lower all-cause and cardiovascular mortality in this analysis. The reason for this paradox is unclear, but one of the hypotheses is that obese patients may have higher metabolic reserve to tolerate advanced heart failure, which is a catabolic state causing cachexia.[53] Also, low levels of B-type natriuretic peptide have been noted in obese patients.[54]

DEMENTIA AND DEPRESSION

Both dementia and heart failure are diseases of old age. There is mounting evidence that heart failure could lead to cognitive impairment in the elderly. This was described even decades ago as "cardiogenic dementia."[55] The possible mechanisms are chronic cerebral hypoperfusion and possible microembolism from the heart. Also, vascular risk factors associated with heart failure are known to cause vascular dementia, which is the second most common form of dementia after Alzheimer dementia. The increased risk of cognitive dysfunction in heart failure was shown in a systematic review that included 17,785 subjects with and without heart failure. The odds ratio for cognitive impairment was 1.62 in patients with heart failure.[56] The prevalence of mild cognitive impairment is much higher in the chronic heart failure population, and was noted in more than 50% of patients.[57] Only scant evidence exists to support that treatment of heart failure may improve cognitive function,[58] and this has to be proved in larger, well-designed studies before the concept is well accepted. Until then, the authors at least recommend regular screening of patients with heart failure for cognitive impairment.

The coprevalence rate of heart failure and depression varies widely depending on the criteria used to diagnose depression and severity of heart failure.[59] In this analysis, clinically significant depression was noted in at least 1 of every 5 patients with heart failure. Many symptoms of heart failure, such as decreased exercise tolerance, sleep disturbances, and weight gain, could lead to depression. Also, neurohormonal activation[60] and chronic inflammation could play a role in the development of depression. In patients with systolic heart failure, major depression was an independent predictor of mortality at 3 months and 1 year. Depressed patients were more than twice as likely to die when compared with patients without depression. Major depression was also associated with increased hospital readmissions.[61] Compliance with diet and medication regimen is extremely important in the management of heart failure, and there is evidence to suggest that depressed patients are 3 times more likely to be noncompliant.[62] Selective serotonin reuptake inhibitors (SSRIs) are clinically preferable to tricyclic antidepressants in patients with heart failure.[63] Although the preliminary results are not encouraging,[64] results from ongoing clinical studies to evaluate the role of SSRIs in the treatment of depression in patients with heart failure is much awaited.[65]

SUMMARY

Multiple comorbidities are common in patients in heart failure. Some of them could contribute to the underlying development of heart failure, whereas others may lead to disease progression and may be associated with poor prognosis. It is not only important to diagnose these comorbid conditions early, but also vital to treat such conditions appropriately, which may have a huge impact on the primary disease itself. This review has covered the common conditions, but there are multiple other comorbidities beyond the scope of this article. The authors advise that physicians should try treating "patients as a whole" instead of treating the specific disease, and this may require multidisciplinary care.

REFERENCES

1. Chobanian AV, Bakris GL, Black HR, et al. The Seventh Report of the Joint National Committee on Prevention, Detection, Evaluation, and Treatment of High Blood Pressure: the JNC 7 report. JAMA 2003;289(19):2560–72.
2. Lloyd-Jones D, Adams R, Carnethon M, et al. Heart disease and stroke statistics—2009 update: a report from the American Heart Association Statistics Committee and Stroke Statistics Subcommittee. Circulation 2009;119(3):480–6.

3. Braunstein JB, Anderson GF, Gerstenblith G, et al. Noncardiac comorbidity increases preventable hospitalizations and mortality among Medicare beneficiaries with chronic heart failure. J Am Coll Cardiol 2003;42(7):1226–33.

4. Wong CY, Chaudhry SI, Desai MM, et al. Trends in comorbidity, disability, and polypharmacy in heart failure. Am J Med 2011;124(2):136–43.

5. Zhang JX, Rathouz PJ, Chin MH. Comorbidity and the concentration of healthcare expenditures in older patients with heart failure. J Am Geriatr Soc 2003; 51(4):476–82.

6. Kannel WB, McGee DL. Diabetes and cardiovascular disease. The Framingham study. JAMA 1979;241(19):2035–8.

7. Stratton IM, Adler AI, Neil HA, et al. Association of glycaemia with macrovascular and microvascular complications of type 2 diabetes (UKPDS 35): prospective observational study. BMJ 2000;321(7258):405–12.

8. Gustafsson I, Brendorp B, Seibaek M, et al. Influence of diabetes and diabetes-gender interaction on the risk of death in patients hospitalized with congestive heart failure. J Am Coll Cardiol 2004;43(5):771–7.

9. Dries DL, Sweitzer NK, Drazner MH, et al. Prognostic impact of diabetes mellitus in patients with heart failure according to the etiology of left ventricular systolic dysfunction. J Am Coll Cardiol 2001;38(2):421–8.

10. Solang L, Malmberg K, Ryden L. Diabetes mellitus and congestive heart failure. Further knowledge needed. Eur Heart J 1999;20(11):789–95.

11. Bell DS. Heart failure in the diabetic patient. Cardiol Clin 2007;25(4):523–38, vi.

12. Eurich DT, McAlister FA, Blackburn DF, et al. Benefits and harms of antidiabetic agents in patients with diabetes and heart failure: systematic review. BMJ 2007; 335(7618):497.

13. Loke YK, Kwok CS, Singh S. Comparative cardiovascular effects of thiazolidinediones: systematic review and meta-analysis of observational studies. BMJ 2011. 342:d1309.

14. Shekelle PG, Rich MW, Morton SC, et al. Efficacy of angiotensin-converting enzyme inhibitors and beta-blockers in the management of left ventricular systolic dysfunction according to race, gender, and diabetic status: a meta-analysis of major clinical trials. J Am Coll Cardiol 2003;41(9):1529–38.

15. Kerr D, MacDonald IA, Heller SR, et al. Beta-adrenoceptor blockade and hypoglycaemia. A randomised, double-blind, placebo controlled comparison of metoprolol CR, atenolol and propranolol LA in normal subjects. Br J Clin Pharmacol 1990;29(6):685–93.

16. Larkin RJ, Atlas SA, Donohue TJ. Spironolactone in patients with heart failure. N Engl J Med 2000;342(2):132–3 [author reply: 133–4].

17. Kannel WB, Ho K, Thom T. Changing epidemiological features of cardiac failure. Br Heart J 1994;72(Suppl 2):S3–9.

18. Levy D, Larson MG, Vasan RS, et al. The progression from hypertension to congestive heart failure. JAMA 1996;275(20):1557–62.

19. SHEP Cooperative Research Group. Prevention of stroke by antihypertensive drug treatment in older persons with isolated systolic hypertension. Final results of the Systolic Hypertension in the Elderly Program (SHEP). JAMA 1991;265(24):3255–64.

20. Dahlof B, Lindholm LH, Hansson L, et al. Morbidity and mortality in the Swedish Trial in Old Patients with Hypertension (STOP-Hypertension). Lancet 1991; 338(8778):1281–5.

21. Levy D, Garrison RJ, Savage DD, et al. Prognostic implications of echocardiographically determined left ventricular mass in the Framingham Heart Study. N Engl J Med 1990;322(22):1561–6.

22. Gradman AH, Alfayoumi F. From left ventricular hypertrophy to congestive heart failure: management of hypertensive heart disease. Prog Cardiovasc Dis 2006; 48(5):326–41.
23. Iriarte MM, Perez Olea J, Sagastagoitia D, et al. Congestive heart failure due to hypertensive ventricular diastolic dysfunction. Am J Cardiol 1995;76(13):43D–7D.
24. Kalantar-Zadeh K, Block G, Horwich T, et al. Reverse epidemiology of conventional cardiovascular risk factors in patients with chronic heart failure. J Am Coll Cardiol 2004;43(8):1439–44.
25. Kjekshus J, Apetrei E, Barrios V, et al. Rosuvastatin in older patients with systolic heart failure. N Engl J Med 2007;357(22):2248–61.
26. Gissi-HF Investigators, Tavazzi L, Maggioni AP, et al. Effect of rosuvastatin in patients with chronic heart failure (the GISSI-HF trial): a randomised, double-blind, placebo-controlled trial. Lancet 2008;372(9645):1231–9.
27. Molyneux SL, Florkowski CM, George PM, et al. Coenzyme Q10: an independent predictor of mortality in chronic heart failure. J Am Coll Cardiol 2008;52(18):1435–41.
28. McMurray JJ, Dunselman P, Wedel H, et al. Coenzyme Q10, rosuvastatin, and clinical outcomes in heart failure: a pre-specified substudy of CORONA (controlled rosuvastatin multinational study in heart failure). J Am Coll Cardiol 2010;56(15): 1196–204.
29. Sinden NJ, Stockley RA. Systemic inflammation and comorbidity in COPD: a result of 'overspill' of inflammatory mediators from the lungs? Review of the evidence. Thorax 2010;65(10):930–6.
30. Bales AC, Sorrentino MJ. Causes of congestive heart failure. Prompt diagnosis may affect prognosis. Postgrad Med 1997;101(1):44–9, 54–6.
31. Maisel AS, Krishnaswamy P, Nowak RM, et al. Rapid measurement of B-type natriuretic peptide in the emergency diagnosis of heart failure. N Engl J Med 2002;347(3):161–7.
32. De Blois J, Simard S, Atar D, et al. COPD predicts mortality in HF: the Norwegian Heart Failure Registry. J Card Fail 2010;16(3):225–9.
33. Hole DJ, Watt GC, Davey-Smith G, et al. Impaired lung function and mortality risk in men and women: findings from the Renfrew and Paisley prospective population study. BMJ 1996;313(7059):711–5 [discussion: 715–6].
34. Godtfredsen NS, Osler M, Vestbo J, et al. Smoking reduction, smoking cessation, and incidence of fatal and non-fatal myocardial infarction in Denmark 1976-1998: a pooled cohort study. J Epidemiol Community Health 2003;57(6):412–6.
35. Salpeter SR, Ormiston TM, Salpeter EE. Cardiovascular effects of beta-agonists in patients with asthma and COPD: a meta-analysis. Chest 2004;125(6):2309–21.
36. Salpeter S, Ormiston T, Salpeter E. Cardioselective beta-blockers for chronic obstructive pulmonary disease. Cochrane Database Syst Rev 2005;(4):CD003566.
37. Kasai T, Bradley TD. Obstructive sleep apnea and heart failure: pathophysiologic and therapeutic implications. J Am Coll Cardiol 2011;57(2):119–27.
38. Gami AS, Pressman G, Caples SM, et al. Association of atrial fibrillation and obstructive sleep apnea. Circulation 2004;110(4):364–7.
39. Gottlieb DJ, Yenokyan G, Newman AB, et al. Prospective study of obstructive sleep apnea and incident coronary heart disease and heart failure: the Sleep Heart Health Study. Circulation 2010;122(4):352–60.
40. Wang H, Parker JD, Newton GE, et al. Influence of obstructive sleep apnea on mortality in patients with heart failure. J Am Coll Cardiol 2007;49(15):1625–31.
41. Javaheri S, Caref EB, Chen E, et al. Sleep apnea testing and outcomes in a large cohort of Medicare beneficiaries with newly diagnosed heart failure. Am J Respir Crit Care Med 2011;183(4):539–46.

42. Bradley TD, Logan AG, Kimoff RJ, et al. Continuous positive airway pressure for central sleep apnea and heart failure. N Engl J Med 2005;353(19):2025–33.

43. Arzt M, Floras JS, Logan AG, et al. Suppression of central sleep apnea by continuous positive airway pressure and transplant-free survival in heart failure: a post hoc analysis of the Canadian Continuous Positive Airway Pressure for Patients with Central Sleep Apnea and Heart Failure Trial (CANPAP). Circulation 2007; 115(25):3173–80.

44. Groenveld HF, Januzzi JL, Damman K, et al. Anemia and mortality in heart failure patients a systematic review and meta-analysis. J Am Coll Cardiol 2008;52(10): 818–27.

45. Tang YD, Katz SD. Anemia in chronic heart failure: prevalence, etiology, clinical correlates, and treatment options. Circulation 2006;113(20):2454–61.

46. Jankowska EA, Rozentryt P, Witkowska A, et al. Iron deficiency: an ominous sign in patients with systolic chronic heart failure. Eur Heart J 2010;31(15):1872–80.

47. Anker SD, Comin Colet J, Filippatos G, et al. Ferric carboxymaltose in patients with heart failure and iron deficiency. N Engl J Med 2009;361(25):2436–48.

48. Ghali JK, Anand IS, Abraham WT, et al. Randomized double-blind trial of darbepoetin alfa in patients with symptomatic heart failure and anemia. Circulation 2008;117(4):526–35.

49. Pfeffer MA, Burdmann EA, Chen CY, et al. A trial of darbepoetin alfa in type 2 diabetes and chronic kidney disease. N Engl J Med 2009;361(21):2019–32.

50. Kenchaiah S, Evans JC, Levy D, et al. Obesity and the risk of heart failure. N Engl J Med 2002;347(5):305–13.

51. Poirier P, Giles TD, Bray GA, et al. Obesity and cardiovascular disease: pathophysiology, evaluation, and effect of weight loss: an update of the 1997 American Heart Association Scientific Statement on Obesity and Heart Disease from the Obesity Committee of the Council on Nutrition, Physical Activity, and Metabolism. Circulation 2006;113(6):898–918.

52. Oreopoulos A, Padwal R, Kalantar-Zadeh K, et al. Body mass index and mortality in heart failure: a meta-analysis. Am Heart J 2008;156(1):13–22.

53. Kenchaiah S, Gaziano JM, Vasan RS. Impact of obesity on the risk of heart failure and survival after the onset of heart failure. Med Clin North Am 2004;88(5):1273–94.

54. Mehra MR, Uber PA, Park MH, et al. Obesity and suppressed B-type natriuretic peptide levels in heart failure. J Am Coll Cardiol 2004;43(9):1590–5.

55. Polidori MC, Marvardi M, Cherubini A, et al. Heart disease and vascular risk factors in the cognitively impaired elderly: implications for Alzheimer's dementia. Aging (Milano) 2001;13(3):231–9.

56. Vogels RL, Scheltens P, Schroeder-Tanka JM, et al. Cognitive impairment in heart failure: a systematic review of the literature. Eur J Heart Fail 2007;9(5):440–9.

57. Zuccala G, Cattel C, Manes-Gravina E, et al. Left ventricular dysfunction: a clue to cognitive impairment in older patients with heart failure. J Neurol Neurosurg Psychiatry 1997;63(4):509–12.

58. Zuccala G, Onder G, Marzetti E, et al. Use of angiotensin-converting enzyme inhibitors and variations in cognitive performance among patients with heart failure. Eur Heart J 2005;26(3):226–33.

59. Rutledge T, Reis VA, Linke SE, et al. Depression in heart failure a meta-analytic review of prevalence, intervention effects, and associations with clinical outcomes. J Am Coll Cardiol 2006;48(8):1527–37.

60. Plotsky PM, Owens MJ, Nemeroff CB. Psychoneuroendocrinology of depression. Hypothalamic-pituitary-adrenal axis. Psychiatr Clin North Am 1998;21(2): 293–307.

61. Jiang W, Alexander J, Christopher E, et al. Relationship of depression to increased risk of mortality and rehospitalization in patients with congestive heart failure. Arch Intern Med 2001;161(15):1849–56.
62. DiMatteo MR, Lepper HS, Croghan TW. Depression is a risk factor for noncompliance with medical treatment: meta-analysis of the effects of anxiety and depression on patient adherence. Arch Intern Med 2000;160(14):2101–7.
63. Jacob S, Sebastian JC, Abraham G. Depression and congestive heart failure: are antidepressants underutilized? Eur J Heart Fail 2003;5(3):399–400.
64. Jiang W, O'Connor C, Silva SG, et al. Safety and efficacy of sertraline for depression in patients with CHF (SADHART-CHF): a randomized, double-blind, placebo-controlled trial of sertraline for major depression with congestive heart failure. Am Heart J 2008;156(3):437–44.
65. Angermann CE, Gelbrich G, Stork S, et al. Rationale and design of a randomised, controlled, multicenter trial investigating the effects of selective serotonin reuptake inhibition on morbidity, mortality and mood in depressed heart failure patients (MOOD-HF). Eur J Heart Fail 2007;9(12):1212–22.

Atrial Fibrillation in Heart Failure

Joel A. Lardizabal, MD[a], Prakash C. Deedwania, MD[b,c],*

KEYWORDS

- Atrial fibrillation • Heart failure • Treatment • Prognosis • Antiarrhythmic therapy
- Catheter ablation • Antithrombotic therapy

KEY POINTS

- Atrial fibrillation (AF) is a marker of worse prognosis in heart failure (HF). The onset of new AF is associated with increased mortality and morbidity in HF.
- Heart rate control is non-inferior to the rhythm control strategy, and remains the first-line approach to treatment in AF with HF.
- Antithrombotic therapy for stroke prophylaxis is required in AF with HF. The availability of new, effective anticoagulants has expanded the therapeutic options.
- Non-pharmacologic strategies, such as catheter ablation procedures, are gaining wide acceptance for the treatment of AF in HF.

BACKGROUND

Chronic heart failure (HF) is a highly prevalent disorder, afflicting about 6 million individuals in the United States, with an incidence of 10 per 1000 population after age 65 years.[1] Nearly 300,000 Americans die from HF annually, and although overall survival has improved over time, mortality remains high, as roughly 50% of patients die within 5 years of diagnosis.[2] The morbidity associated with HF is also substantial, as it accounts for approximately 1 million inpatient hospitalizations and 3.5 million ambulatory care visits each year, at an estimated cost of $35 billion.[3] Mitigating the enormous public health burden exerted by HF is of paramount importance, and key to this is the recognition and management of its associated conditions or risk factors, which include atrial fibrillation (AF).

Chronic AF is the most predominant of the clinically relevant arrhythmias. The overall prevalence of AF is considerably higher in patients with HF, and has been reported to be as high as 25%.[4] AF and chronic HF (CHF) can perpetuate each other. Both

Disclosure: The authors have no relevant disclosure related to this submitted work.
[a] Division of Cardiology, Department of Medicine, University of California-San Francisco (Fresno-MEP), 155 North Fresno Street, Fresno, CA 93701, USA; [b] School of Medicine, University of California-San Francisco, San Francisco, CA, USA; [c] Cardiology Division, Veterans Affairs Central California System, VACCHS Medical Center, 2515 East Clinton Avenue, Fresno, CA 93703, USA
* Corresponding author.
E-mail address: deed@fresno.ucsf.edu

conditions share common risk factors, such as advanced age, hypertension, diabetes mellitus, coronary artery disease, and valvular heart disease. There is also evidence of a more complex relationship between HF and AF that may be independent of these mutual predisposing factors. Because of the complex interaction between AF and HF, it is useful to review the prognostic relationship between these 2 conditions, pathophysiologic mechanisms, and appropriate therapeutic strategies for their management.

PROGNOSTIC RELATIONSHIP BETWEEN AF AND HF

CHF is the strongest predictor for the development of AF, with up to a sixfold increase in risk seen in the Framingham Study.[5] The prevalence of AF in the setting of preexisting HF increases with worsening HF symptoms: 4% in functional class I, up to 27% in functional class II to III, and 50% in functional class IV patients.[6] Even with optimal medical therapy, the onset of AF is often accompanied by cardiac decompensation and functional class deterioration in patients with HF. Hemodynamic alterations that can be observed shortly after AF onset include marked reductions in peak oxygen consumption and cardiac index, as well as increases in the severity of valvular regurgitation and cardiac chamber dimensions.[7]

AF has significant prognostic implications in patients with HF. A retrospective analysis of the Studies of Left ventricular Dysfunction (SOLVD)[8] involving more than 4200 patients with symptomatic and asymptomatic HF, showed that the presence of AF was associated with significant increases in the risks of total mortality by 32%, pump-failure death by 48%, and HF hospitalization by 38%. A similar observation was noted from the analysis of data from the Candesartan in Heart failure-Assessment of Reduction in Mortality and Morbidity (CHARM)[9] trial, which enrolled 7600 patients with symptomatic HF, 15% of whom had AF. In patients with low systolic function, AF was associated with a 29% higher risk of mortality or HF hospitalization. In those with preserved systolic function, the relative risk of adverse events is even higher at 72%. A meta-analysis of 16 studies that evaluated nearly 54,000 patients with HF showed a 40% increased risk for total mortality if AF was present.[10] The increase in adverse outcomes associated with AF was observed in both preserved and impaired ventricular HF types.

The mere presence of AF per se, while serving as a marker of poor outcomes, may not necessarily affect the prognosis of patients with HF in a direct and independent manner. For example, post hoc analysis of data from the Veterans Affairs Vasodilator-Heart Failure Trials (V-HeFT),[11] which enrolled more than 1300 patients with mild to moderate HF, found that the rates of mortality, hospitalization, and other adverse events in patients with AF were no different from those in sinus rhythm. Similarly, in severe HF, AF has not been shown to be independently associated with adverse outcomes in the Prospective Randomized Study of Ibopamine on Mortality and Efficacy (PRIME)[12] study, which enrolled more than 400 patients with advanced chronic HF.

The prognostic role of AF in HF was later clarified in the post hoc analysis of data from the Carvedilol Or Metoprolol European Trial (COMET), which enrolled more than 3000 patients with symptomatic systolic HF, 20% of whom had AF at baseline. Univariate analysis showed that patients who were in AF on baseline electrocardiogaphy had significantly higher risks of all-cause and cardiovascular mortality and hospitalization rates over a 5-year period (**Fig. 1**). After adjustment for patient-related variables (eg, age and gender), however, the presence of AF at baseline was no longer independently associated with mortality. Serial electrocardiography was performed

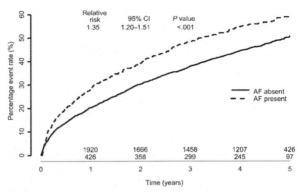

Fig. 1. Cardiovascular mortality or hospitalization for worsening heart failure by baseline atrial fibrillation in the COMET trial.

throughout the COMET follow-up period to screen for subsequent development of AF. Of the nearly 2500 patients who were in sinus rhythm at baseline, 580 developed new-onset AF during the study. In this subset of patients, new-onset AF was an independent predictor of subsequent all-cause mortality and remained so regardless of treatment and changes in functional class over time.[13] In summary, although preexisting chronic AF has not been definitively shown to independently affect the mortality or morbidity rates in patients with HF, the onset of new AF is certainly associated with adverse outcomes in chronic HF.

PATHOPHYSIOLOGIC MECHANISMS

Under normal circumstances, atrial systole may contribute up to 25% of the cardiac output. In the setting of ventricular dysfunction, the atrial contribution to the total cardiac output could be as high as 50%. The onset of AF abolishes the "atrial kick" leading to reductions in cardiac output, peak oxygen uptake, and exercise tolerance.[14,15] When the failing heart is subjected to these adverse hemodynamic conditions, cardiac decompensation occurs.

In addition, the onset of AF also decreases cardiac output and worsens HF through other mechanisms. AF may cause valvular regurgitation, which causes reduction in forward blood flow. Rapid ventricular rates during periods of uncontrolled AF lead to inadequate ventricle filling time and decrease in stroke volume.[16–18] An irregular ventricular response, in itself and independent of heart rate, causes a drop in cardiac output, increase in pulmonary wedge pressure, and elevation of right atrial pressure.[19]

In patients with normal baseline ventricular function, the chronic rapid heart rates associated with AF can produce a distinct, reversible type of severe biventricular HF called "tachycardia-induced cardiomyopathy." On a hemodynamic level, the incessant tachycardia seen in AF impairs myocardial compliance and shortens the ventricle filling times, leading to a reduction in cardiac output and subsequent development of symptomatic HF. Higher heart rates and longer tachycardia duration generally lead to more severe HF. Ultrastructural cardiac remodeling occurs, characterized by cytoskeletal alteration, matrix metalloproteinase disruption, depletion of high-energy stores, and induction of abnormal calcium handling. The negative remodeling process is also accompanied by neurohormonal derangements, such as increased sympathetic response and activation of the renin-angiotensin system (RAS).[20–22]

In patients with HF with sinus rhythm at baseline, the ultrastuctural and neurohormonal aberrations that are induced by cardiac dysfunction produce a favorable substrate for the development and maintenance of atrial and ventricular arrhythmias, including AF. High intracardiac volumes and pressures in HF can cause mechanical stretching of the atria, which is associated with shortening of the atrial refractory period, prolongation of atrial conduction times, increased frequency of interatrial conduction blocks, and heightened atrial irritability.[23,24] Stimulation of the sympathetic nervous system and high catecholamine levels that are features of chronic HF not only increase the ventricular rate response in AF, but may cause abnormalities of atrial action potentials and automaticity that can trigger arrhythmogenesis as well.[25] Parasympathetic hyperinnervation is part of a complex autonomic remodeling process seen in HF, and contributes significantly to the maintenance of AF.[26] HF is also accosted by activation of the RAS system and increased angiotensin-II expression, which induce atrial interstitial fibrosis, creating areas of slowed conduction and heterogeneity in repolarization that serve as substrates for AF generation.[25,27] In the failing atrium, profound calcium dysregulation and ion channel remodeling within the atrial cardiomyocyte enhance arrhythmogenesis and promote triggered activity in AF.[28]

THERAPEUTIC STRATEGIES: RATE VERSUS RHYTHM CONTROL OF AF IN HF

Although most of the landmark trials on AF therapy have shown that the therapeutic strategy of rhythm-control (conversion to and maintenance of sinus rhythm using antiarrhythmic agents) generally had no clinical advantage over that of simple rate control (AF is not actively converted to sinus rhythm, but heart rate [HR] is maintained at a specified target range), retrospective analyses of early major trials in HF pointed toward favorable outcomes with rhythm control.

For example, 103 patients with HF with baseline AF who enrolled in the Congestive Heart Failure: Survival Trial of Antiarrhythmic Therapy (CHF-STAT)[29] were randomized to treatment with either amiodarone or placebo. Of those treated with amiodarone, 31% converted to sinus rhythm. After 4 years of follow-up, significantly lower mortality rate was noted in patients with HF with baseline AF who subsequently converted to sinus rhythm on amiodarone compared with nonresponders. Also, subgroup analysis of data from 261 patients with AF with mild to moderate HF who enrolled in the Rate-Control Efficacy in Permanent Atrial Fibrillation (RACE)[30] trial showed improved survival, less frequent HF hospitalization, and lower adverse events with rhythm control compared with rate control. A similar observation was seen in the post hoc analysis of patients with HF enrolled in the Danish Investigations of Arrhythmia and Mortality on Dofetilide (DIAMOND),[31] 506 of whom had baseline AF. The study showed that the restoration and maintenance of sinus rhythm in patients with HF with AF was associated with significant reductions in mortality and hospitalization rates.

A small prospective study (CAFÉ-II)[32] randomized 61 patients with chronic HF and persistent AF into either rhythm-control or rate-control treatment approaches. After 1 year of follow-up, the trial found improved ventricular function and better quality of life in the rhythm-control group. The clinical benefit of rhythm control, however, was not demonstrated in the landmark Atrial Fibrillation in Congestive Heart Failure (AF-CHF) trial.[33] In this study, nearly 1400 patients with AF and concomitant HF were randomized to either rhythm-control or rate-control strategies. After 3 years of follow-up, the trial found no difference in the rates of mortality and major cardiovascular events in either group (**Fig. 2**). Probably contributing to the lack of net clinical

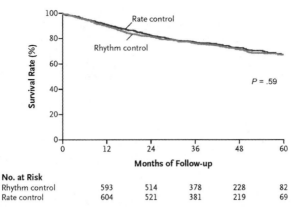

Fig. 2. A comparison of Kaplan-Meier estimates of death from cardiovascular causes in patients with atrial fibrillation and heart failure treated with rhythm-control or rate-control strategies in the AF-CHF trial.

benefit of the rhythm-control approach is the suboptimal efficacy and relative toxicity of the antiarrhythmic drugs that were used.

RATE-CONTROL APPROACHES
Pharmacologic Rate Control

Beta adrenergic blocking agents are the preferred HR-modulating drugs for AF because of their established cardioprotective effects in the setting of HF. Bisoprolol, metoprolol succinate, and carvedilol have demonstrated mortality benefit in HF,[34] and have been shown to provide effective rate control in patients with AF with HF. The current guidelines also recommend digoxin as a first-line agent in the control of HR in patients with AF with systolic dysfunction and HF.[35] In the presence of adequate beta blockade, digoxin does not appear to be significantly effective; however, in cases when adequate doses of beta blocker are not tolerated or contraindicated, digoxin should be considered the first-line therapy.

Strict Versus Lenient Rate Control

Traditionally, treatment targets for HR for AF have been defined to range between 60 and 80/min at rest and 80 to 110/min with moderate exercise. These arbitrary goals are often difficult to accomplish, especially in patients with HF, and have been recently challenged by the results of the Rate Control Efficacy in Permanent Atrial Fibrillation (RACE-II) trial.[36] The study enrolled more than 600 patients with AF, 10% of whom had previous hospitalization for HF, who were randomized to either lenient (target resting HR <110/min) or strict rate control (target HR <80/min at rest, <110/min on moderate exercise). After 3 years of follow-up, there was no significant difference seen in the composite rates of death, HF hospitalization, or major cardiovascular events between the 2 groups (**Fig. 3**). However, specific data on patients with HF were not released and the long-term effect of the lenient rate control approach on systolic function was not evaluated, so the results of the RACE-II trial cannot be extrapolated to the general HF population with AF at this time.

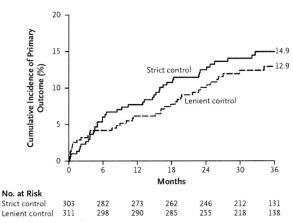

Fig. 3. Kaplan-Meier estimates of the cumulative incidence of major adverse cardiac events in patients with atrial fibrillation treated with either strict or lenient rate-control strategies in the RACE-II trial.

Target Heart Rate in CHF

The optimal HR goal for HF treatment has not yet been defined, although previous studies have highlighted the prognostic role of HR in patients with HF. For example, post hoc analyses of the CIBIS-I (Cardiac Insufficiency Bisoprolol Study)[37] and COMET[38] found that HR assessed a few months after initiating beta-blocker therapy had an independent prognostic value for subsequent outcomes in patients with HF. Recent data suggest that HR may be a suitable modifiable target in HF therapy. Subgroup analysis of the BEAUTIFUL trial (Morbidity-Mortality Evaluation of the I_f Inhibitor Ivabradine in Patients With Coronary Disease and Left Ventricular Dysfunction),[39] involving nearly 5500 patients with systolic dysfunction, found that those with resting HR above 70/min had a 34% higher risk of mortality and a 53% higher frequency of HF hospitalization compared with patients with resting HR below 70/min.

Subsequently, a rate-control strategy in patients with HF was tested in the Systolic Heart Failure Treatment with the I_f inhibitor Ivabradine Trial (SHIFT)[40] using the novel selective sinus-node inhibitor ivabradine. In this trial, more than 6500 patients with HF (8% of whom had AF) with resting HR above 70/min were randomized to treatment with either placebo or ivabradine, dose adjusted to maintain HR between 50 and 60/min. After nearly 2 years of follow-up, the study showed that HR reduction with ivabradine was associated with a 26% reduction in HF deaths and 24% decrease in hospitalization for worsening HF. Whether or not the results are applicable to the general AF population with HF remains unclear. Furthermore, it is important to note that ivabradine, which primarily works by its action on I_f channels in the sinus node, has no effect on atrioventricular (AV) nodal conduction and, as such, does not appear to be useful in controlling ventricular rate in patients with AF.

Nonpharmacologic Rate Control

If drug therapy is unsuccessful or not tolerated, nonpharmacologic approaches to AF rate control can be performed, such as transcatheter ablation of the AV node or His bundle or modification of the AV nodal conduction. In transcatheter AV node ablation, a complete heart block is created with the use of direct current or radiofrequency energy, electrically separating the atria from the ventricles. A permanent pacing device is subsequently implanted to adequately control the ventricular rate.[41] Alternatively, radiofrequency energy can be used to modify, rather than completely abolish, AV nodal conduction. Ablation of one of the 2 electrical pathways within the AV node can reduce the number of impulses that successfully reach the infranodal conduction system and the ventricles. This precludes the need for permanent pacemaker implantation, although procedural success rate is lower compared with complete AV node ablation.[42]

AV nodal ablation could have a favorable effect in patients with HF on cardiac resynchronization therapy (CRT) and concomitant AF. In this group of patients, a small study found lower rates of mortality and adverse outcomes, as well as greater functional class improvement, in those who underwent AV nodal ablation compared with those given drug therapy for AF rate control.[43] However, larger randomized trials are required to confirm this observation before this approach is considered.

RHYTHM CONTROL STRATEGY
Pharmacologic Rhythm Control

Although in general, rhythm control is not superior to simple rate control in patients with HF with AF, this approach may be worthwhile in individuals who are symptomatic during AF episodes even if HR is adequately controlled. For this indication, amiodarone or dofetilide may be used for pharmacologic rhythm control of AF in the setting of HF. If concurrent coronary disease or significant left ventricle hypertrophy is present, however, dofetilide is contraindicated, leaving amiodarone as the sole agent of choice in these cases.[34] Although amiodarone is a well-tested therapy that has been used in a number of clinical trials, including in patients with HF, it does have its limitations because of significant drug-drug interactions (especially with polypharmacy in patients with HF) and HF-related alterations in the volume of distribution and overall drug metabolism and elimination.

Dronedarone

The relative dearth of safer and more tolerable antiarrhythmic drugs in AF therapy has led to the development of the novel agent dronedarone, a derivative of amiodarone that has a shorter half-life and is devoid of iodine moiety to reduce toxicity. In the general AF population, the incidence of major adverse effects with dronedarone was similar to placebo and 20% lower compared with amiodarone.[44] In patients with advanced HF, however, the Antiarrhythmic Trial with Dronedarone in Moderate to Severe CHF Evaluating Morbidity Decrease (ANDROMEDA)[45] found a twofold excess in mortality with dronedarone compared with placebo, primarily because of worsening HF, prompting the early termination of this study after just 2 months of clinical follow-up. On the other hand, the ATHENA trial (A Placebo-Controlled, Double-Blind, Parallel Arm Trial To Assess the Efficacy of Dronedarone 400 mg Bid for the Prevention of Cardiovascular Hospitalization or Death from Any Cause in Patients With Atrial Fibrillation/Atrial Flutter) enrolled more than 4600 patients with AF, 21% of whom had HF with functional class II or III symptoms. The study found that dronedarone therapy was associated with significant reductions in morbidity and mortality in patients with AF.[46] The seemingly conflicting findings of these 2 trials have led some to hypothesize that dronedarone possibly increases mortality among patients with advanced and recently decompensated HF, but reduces those same adverse events in patients with less severe heart failure. Currently, the drug carries a Black Box Warning listing severely symptomatic or recently decompensated HF as a contraindication to dronedarone therapy.

Nonpharmacologic Rhythm Control

The track record of current antiarrhythmic drug therapy is rather disappointing. On the contrary, the alternative nonpharmacologic interventions that are available for the maintenance of sinus rhythm in patients with AF and HF have been promising. The Cox-Maze procedure, a major open-heart surgical technique, involves placing multiple incisions within the atria to interrupt reentry pathways. It has an excellent efficacy in the general AF population (90% freedom from AF at 10 years), with a 1.4% early operative mortality rate.[47] Although often avoided in high-risk patients with HF, the Cox-Maze procedure, when performed in the setting of severe systolic dysfunction, was associated with significant improvements in ejection fraction, functional class, and quality of life. The efficacy of this surgical procedure remains high at 86% without increasing operative risk in patients with HF.[48] With recent modifications in surgical technique, the procedure is now being performed in a simpler, minimally invasive fashion (eg, mini-Maze), resulting in less incidence of perioperative morbidity while achieving comparable efficacy as the classic Cox-Maze procedure.[49]

Transcatheter AF ablation is a safer and less invasive alternative to the surgical approaches. Like the Cox-Maze procedure, the transcatheter approach aims to interrupt reentry pathways and isolate the pulmonary veins and arrhythmogenic AF foci by placing multiple ablation lines within the atria. It has been shown to be safe and effective in patients with HF, although some operators are still reluctant to perform the procedure in these patients because of technical concerns. The PABA-CHF (Pulmonary Vein Antrum Isolation vs AV Node Ablation With Bi-Ventricular Pacing for Treatment of Atrial Fibrillation in Patients With Congestive Heart Failure)[50] trial randomized more than 80 patients with drug-resistant AF and symptomatic systolic HF to either transcatheter pulmonary vein isolation (PVI) or AV nodal ablation with permanent pacing. After 6 months of follow-up, patients who underwent PVI had significantly higher improvements in ejection fraction, functional capacity, and quality of life. Freedom from AF was achieved in 78% of patients after PVI, with no periprocedural deaths reported.

The popularity of transcatheter AF ablation has dramatically increased over the past few years, and is now considered a part of the standard therapies for patients with AF who have failed drug therapy. The large, multicenter, randomized CASTLE-AF (Catheter Ablation vs Standard Conventional Treatment in Patients With Left Ventricular Dysfunction and Atrial Fibrillation) trial is currently ongoing, with the objective of comparing transcatheter AF ablation versus conventional medical treatment in terms of mortality and morbidity in patients with AF and HF. Until then, ablation techniques remain as second-line alternatives to pharmacologic therapy in the rhythm-control approach to patients with AF with HF.[51]

NON-ANTIARRHYTHMIC THERAPY

Non-antiarrhythmic therapeutic alternatives to the conventional antiarrhythmic drugs in AF management have been explored, but their clinical utility is still a subject of debate. Retrospective and epidemiologic data suggest that statins, omega-3 fatty acids, antioxidants, anti-inflammatory agents, and ranozaline may favorably alter the natural course of AF by modulating the underlying structural, electrophysiologic, and neurohormonal substrates that fuel atrial arrhythmogenesis.[52] Data from small-scale studies and experimental models suggest that these alternative therapies may be of benefit in the setting of HF as well.[53–55] However, the clinical efficacy of these therapeutic alternatives for patients with AF and HF has never been corroborated in large randomized trials, and their role in actual practice remains undefined.

The RAS inhibitors have been the mainstay of HF pharmacotherapy owing to their well-established mortality and morbidity benefit. This class of non-antiarrhythmic agents has recently attracted interest because of its potential role in AF management. A meta-analysis of 23 randomized trials involving more than 87,000 patients who were treated with RAS blockers showed a 33% reduction in the risk of AF in those who received angiotensin-converting enzyme inhibitors or angiotensin receptor blockers (ARBs). Patients with HF appeared to derive the most benefit from these agents.[56] However, these observations were not substantiated by the results of the recently concluded ACTIVE-I (Atrial Fibrillation Clopidogrel Trial With Irbesartan for Prevention of Vascular Events) trial,[57] which randomized more than 9000 high-risk patients with AF (32% of whom had HF) to treatment with either placebo or the ARB irbesartan. After 4 years of follow-up, the study found no difference in the composite rates of cardiovascular events, hospitalizations, mortality, and stroke between groups, implying that RAS blockade does not provide additional therapeutic benefit in patients with AF. Of note, the study found a lower incidence of HF hospitalizations in the treatment arm. Specific data on the subset of patients with HF have not been released, but RAS inhibitors remain an integral part in the management of these patients even though the effect on AF has not been convincing.

ANTITHROMBOTIC THERAPY

HF is a major risk factor for thromboembolic events in AF, and, thus, antithrombotic therapy is required in these patients whether a rhythm-control or rate-control treatment approach is chosen. Oral anticoagulation with warfarin has been the mainstay of stroke prophylaxis in AF. Patients with AF with HF who do not have any of the other CHADS2 risk factors (eg, hypertension, age older than 75 years, diabetes, and stroke) may be given aspirin as an alternative, although oral anticoagulation is preferred.[34]

Warfarin, although highly effective, has many limitations, including slow onset of action, significant drug-drug and food-drug interactions, and narrow therapeutic window. This is further complicated by the pharmacokinetic and pharmacodynamic alterations that are associated with HF. A reduction in the volume of distribution and impairment in drug clearance may result from HF-related end-organ hypoperfusion, as well as congestion of the liver and gut.[58] Thus, maintenance of optimal anticoagulation is particularly challenging with warfarin in patients with HF.

Dabigatran

Over the past decade, more effective and efficient alternatives to warfarin have been explored, which led to the emergence of dabigatran, a direct oral thrombin inhibitor that has a rapid onset of action, less food and drug interaction, and more predictable anticoagulation response, which permits fixed dosing without the need for coagulation monitoring. The clinical efficacy and safety of dabigatran was evaluated in the RE-LY (Randomized Evaluation of Long-Term Anticoagulation Therapy)[59] trial, which randomized more than 18,000 high-risk patients with AF into treatment with either warfarin or dabigatran (in 2 separate dosing arms of 110 mg or 150 mg twice daily). After 2 years of follow-up, the study found that low-dose dabigatran had similar antithrombotic efficacy in preventing thromboembolic events but had significantly lower rates of bleeding compared with warfarin. High-dose dabigatran, on the other hand, was associated with a significant 34% lowering of embolic events compared with warfarin without increasing bleeding risk (**Fig. 4**). As such, dabigatran is now considered an important alternative to warfarin, and the practice guidelines have been recently updated to reflect the addition of dabigatran as a first-line option for anticoagulation for high-risk patients with AF, which include those with HF.[60]

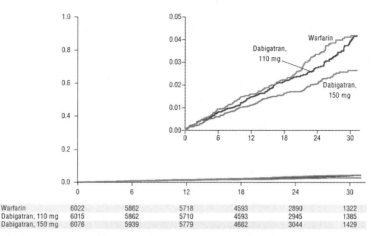

Fig. 4. Cumulative hazard rates of stroke or systemic embolism in patients with atrial fibrillation treated with warfarin or dabigatran in the RE-LY trial.

Dual Antiplatelet Therapy

In patients who are unsuitable for warfarin therapy, the ACTIVE-A trial, which enrolled more than 7500 high-risk patients with AF, found that dual antiplatelet therapy using combination aspirin and clopidogrel was 28% more effective than aspirin monotherapy in preventing stroke. There was, however, a higher incidence of major bleeding events seen with dual antiplatelet therapy. The revised AF guidelines point out that dual antiplatelet therapy may be considered in patients who cannot safely sustain anticoagulation using warfarin.[51] In those who are otherwise candidates for oral anticoagulation, the ACTIVE-W trial[61] has clearly demonstrated the superiority of warfarin over combination aspirin-clopidogrel in the prevention of thromboembolic events.

SUMMARY

HF and AF are highly prevalent disorders that exert tremendous burden to the health care system. Presence of chronic AF is a marker of worse prognosis in patients with CHF, and the onset of new AF in those with chronic HF is associated with increased morbidity and mortality. This may be because of the numerous hemodynamic impairments associated with the arrhythmia, as well as the accompanying adverse ultrastructural and neurohormonal processes that ultimately lead to cardiac decompensation. Pharmacologic rhythm control has been shown to have no clinical advantage over simple rate control in patients with AF, including those with HF. The use of the new, relatively safer antiarrhythmic agent dronedarone has also resulted in net harm in the setting of HF. A lenient approach to HR is now considered a viable strategy in the general AF population, although its safety in patients with HF is still unclear. Improvements in procedural techniques have resulted in increased efficacy and safety of the surgical and interventional approaches (eg, Maze procedure and transcatheter AF ablation/PVI) to the maintenance of sinus rhythm in patients with AF with HF. As such, their popularity has recently skyrocketed. Until more data establishing their superiority are available, however, these invasive procedures remain as alternative therapies to the first-line pharmacologic rhythm control. Patients with HF are at high risk for AF-related systemic thromboembolic events. The emergence of dabigatran as a more practical alternative to warfarin in AF thromboprophylaxis has been a cause of excitement recently. All of these advances in drug development, nonpharmacologic modalities, and therapeutic strategies have been instrumental in reducing the negative impact of AF and HF.

REFERENCES

1. National Heart, Lung, and Blood Institute. NHLBI Fiscal Year 2009 Factbook. Maryland (US): National Institutes of Health; 2009.
2. American Heart Association Heart Disease, Stroke Statistics Writing Group. Executive summary: heart disease and stroke statistics—2011 update: a report from the American Heart Association. Circulation 2011;123(4):459–63.
3. Lloyd-Jones D, Larson M, Leip E, et al. Lifetime risk for developing congestive heart failure: the Framingham Heart Study. Circulation 2002;106:3068.
4. Cleland JG, Swedberg K, Follath F, et al. The EuroHeart Failure survey programme—a survey on the quality of care among patients with heart failure in Europe. Part 1: patient characteristics and diagnosis. Eur Heart J 2003;24: 442–63.
5. Benjamin EJ, Levy D, Vaziri SM, et al. Independent risk factors for atrial fibrillation in a population-based cohort: the Framingham Heart Study. JAMA 1994;271(11):840–4.
6. Deedwania PC, Lardizabal JA. Atrial fibrillation in heart failure: a comprehensive review. Am J Med 2010;123(3):198–204.
7. Pozzoli M, Cioffi G, Traversi E, et al. Predictors of primary atrial fibrillation and concomitant clinical and hemodynamic changes in patients with chronic heart failure: a prospective study in 344 patients with baseline sinus rhythm. J Am Coll Cardiol 1998;32(1):197–204.
8. Dries DL, Exner DV, Gersh BJ, et al. Atrial fibrillation is associated with an increased risk for mortality and heart failure progression in patients with asymptomatic and symptomatic left ventricular systolic dysfunction: a retrospective analysis of the SOLVD trials. J Am Coll Cardiol 1998;32(3):695–703.
9. Olsson LG, Swedberg K, Ducharme A, et al. Atrial fibrillation and risk of clinical events in chronic heart failure with and without left ventricular systolic dysfunction: results from the Candesartan in Heart failure-Assessment of Reduction in Mortality and morbidity (CHARM) program. J Am Coll Cardiol 2006;47(10): 1997–2004.
10. Mamas MA, Caldwell JC, Chacko S, et al. A meta-analysis of the prognostic significance of atrial fibrillation in chronic heart failure. Eur J Heart Fail 2009; 11(7):676–83.
11. Carson PE, Johnson GR, Dunkman WB, et al. The influence of atrial fibrillation on prognosis in mild to moderate heart failure. The V-HeFT Studies. The V-HeFT VA Cooperative Studies Group. Circulation 1993;87(Suppl 6):VI102–10.
12. Crijns HJ, Tjeerdsma G, de Kam PJ, et al. Prognostic value of the presence and development of atrial fibrillation in patients with advanced chronic heart failure. Eur Heart J 2000;21(15):1238–45.
13. Swedberg K, Olsson LG, Charlesworth A, et al. Prognostic relevance of atrial fibrillation in patients with chronic heart failure on long-term treatment with beta-blockers: results from COMET. Eur Heart J 2005;26(13):1303–8.
14. Leonard JJ, Shaver J, Thompson M. Left atrial transport function. Trans Am Clin Climatol Assoc 1981;92:133–41.
15. Rahimtoola SH, Ehsani A, Sinno MZ, et al. Left atrial transport function in myocardial infarction. Importance of its booster pump function. Am J Med 1975;59(5): 686–94.

16. Raymond RJ, Lee AJ, Messineo FC, et al. Cardiac performance early after cardioversion from atrial fibrillation. Am Heart J 1998;136(3):435–42.
17. Shite J, Yokota Y, Yokoyama M. Heterogeneity and time course of improvement in cardiac function after cardioversion of chronic atrial fibrillation: assessment of serial echocardiographic indices. Br Heart J 1993;70(2):154–9.
18. Pardaens K, Van Cleemput J, Vanhaecke J, et al. Atrial fibrillation is associated with a lower exercise capacity in male chronic heart failure patients. Heart 1997;78:564–8.
19. Clark DM, Plumb VJ, Epstein AE, et al. Hemodynamic effects of an irregular sequence of ventricular cycle lengths during atrial fibrillation. J Am Coll Cardiol 1997;30(4):1039–45.
20. Shinbane JS, Wood MA, Jensen DN, et al. Tachycardia-induced cardiomyopathy: a review of animal models and clinical studies. J Am Coll Cardiol 1997;29(4): 709–15.
21. Byrne MJ, Raman JS, Alferness CA, et al. An ovine model of tachycardia-induced degenerative dilated cardiomyopathy and heart failure with prolonged onset. J Card Fail 2002;8(2):108–15.
22. Nerheim P, Birger-Botkin S, Piracha L, et al. Heart failure and sudden death in patients with tachycardia-induced cardiomyopathy and recurrent tachycardia. Circulation 2004;110:247–52.
23. Solti F, Vecsey T, Kékesi V, et al. The effect of atrial dilatation on the genesis of atrial arrhythmias. Cardiovasc Res 1989;23(10):882–6.
24. Eijsbouts SC, Majidi M, van Zandvoort M, et al. Effects of acute atrial dilation on heterogeneity in conduction in the isolated rabbit heart. J Cardiovasc Electrophysiol 2003;14:269–78.
25. Boyden PA, Tilley LP, Albala A, et al. Mechanisms for atrial arrhythmias associated with cardiomyopathy: a study of feline hearts with primary myocardial disease. Circulation 1984;69:1036–47.
26. Ng J, Villuendas R, Cokic I, et al. Autonomic remodeling in the left atrium and pulmonary veins in heart failure—creation of a dynamic substrate for atrial fibrillation. Circ Arrhythm Electrophysiol 2011;4(3):388–96.
27. Li D, Shinagawa K, Pang L, et al. Effects of angiotensin-converting enzyme inhibition on the development of the atrial fibrillation substrate in dogs with ventricular tachypacing—induced congestive heart failure. Circulation 2001; 104:2608.
28. Yeh Y, Wakili R, Qi X, et al. Calcium-handling abnormalities underlying atrial arrhythmogenesis and contractile dysfunction in dogs with congestive heart failure. Circ Arrhythm Electrophysiol 2008;1:93–102.
29. Deedwania PC, Singh BN, Ellenbogen K, et al. Spontaneous conversion and maintenance of sinus rhythm by amiodarone in patients with heart failure and atrial fibrillation: observations from the Veterans Affairs congestive heart failure survival trial of antiarrhythmic therapy (CHF-STAT). Circulation 1998;98(23): 2574–9.
30. Hagens VE, Crijns HJ, Van Veldhuisen DJ, et al. Rate control versus rhythm control for patients with persistent atrial fibrillation with mild to moderate heart failure: results from the RAte Control versus Electrical cardioversion (RACE) study. Am Heart J 2005;149(6):1106–11.
31. Pedersen OD, Bagger H, Keller N, et al. Efficacy of dofetilide in the treatment of atrial fibrillation-flutter in patients with reduced left ventricular function: a Danish investigations of arrhythmia and mortality on dofetilide (DIAMOND) substudy. Circulation 2001;104(3):292–6.

32. Shelton RJ, Clark AL, Goode K, et al. A randomised, controlled study of rate versus rhythm control in patients with chronic atrial fibrillation and heart failure (CAFE-II). Heart 2009;95(11):924–30.

33. Roy D, Talajic M, Nattel S, et al. Rhythm control versus rate control for atrial fibrillation and heart failure. N Engl J Med 2008;358(25):2667–77.

34. Domanski MJ, Krause-Steinrauf H, Massie BM, et al. A comparative analysis of the results from 4 trials of beta-blocker therapy for heart failure: BEST, CIBIS-II, MERIT-HF, and COPERNICUS. J Card Fail 2003;9(5):354–63.

35. Fuster V, Rydén LE, Cannom DS, et al. ACC/AHA/ESC 2006 guidelines for the management of patients with atrial fibrillation. Circulation 2006;114(7):e257–354.

36. Van Gelder IC, Groenveld HF, Crijns HJ, et al. Lenient versus strict rate control in patients with atrial fibrillation. N Engl J Med 2010;362(15):1363–73.

37. Lechat P, Escolano S, Golmard JL, et al. Prognostic value of bisoprolol-induced hemodynamic effects in heart failure during the Cardiac Insufficiency Bisoprolol Study (CIBIS). Circulation 1997;96:2197–205.

38. Metra M, Torp-Pedersen C, Swedberg K, et al. Influence of heart rate, blood pressure, and beta-blocker dose on outcome and the differences in outcome between carvedilol and metoprolol tartrate in patients with chronic heart failure: results from the COMET trial. Eur Heart J 2005;26(21):2259–68.

39. Fox K, Ford I, Steg PG, et al. Heart rate as a prognostic risk factor in patients with coronary artery disease and left-ventricular systolic dysfunction (BEAUTIFUL): a subgroup analysis of a randomised controlled trial. Lancet 2008;372(9641): 817–21.

40. Swedberg K, Komajda M, Böhm M, et al. Ivabradine and outcomes in chronic heart failure (SHIFT): a randomised placebo-controlled study. Lancet 2010; 376(9744):875–85.

41. Olgin JE, Scheinman MM. Comparison of high energy direct current and radiofrequency catheter ablation of the atrioventricular junction. J Am Coll Cardiol 1993; 21(3):557–64.

42. Williamson BD, Man KC, Daoud E, et al. Radiofrequency catheter modification of atrioventricular conduction to control the ventricular rate during atrial fibrillation. N Engl J Med 1994;331(14):910–7.

43. Dong K, Shen WK, Powell BD, et al. Atrioventricular nodal ablation predicts survival benefit in patients with atrial fibrillation receiving cardiac resynchronization therapy. Heart Rhythm 2010;7(9):1240–5.

44. Lardizabal JA, Huang G, Deedwania PC. Modern pharmacologic strategies in the management of atrial fibrillation. J Innov Card Rhythm Management 2011;2: 1–9.

45. Køber L, Torp-Pedersen C, McMurray JJ, et al. Increased mortality after dronedarone therapy for severe heart failure. N Engl J Med 2008;358(25):2678–87.

46. ATHENA Investigators. Effect of dronedarone on cardiovascular events in atrial fibrillation. N Engl J Med 2009;360(7):668–78.

47. Gaynor SL, Schuessler RB, Bailey MS, et al. Surgical treatment of atrial fibrillation: predictors of late recurrence. J Thorac Cardiovasc Surg 2005;129(1):104–11.

48. Ad N, Henry L, Hunt S. The impact of surgical ablation in patients with low ejection fraction, heart failure, and atrial fibrillation. Eur J Cardiothorac Surg 2011; 40(1):70–6.

49. Cui YQ, Sun LB, Li Y, et al. Intraoperative modified Cox mini-maze procedure for long-standing persistent atrial fibrillation. Ann Thorac Surg 2008;85(4):1283–9.

50. Khan MN, Jaïs P, Cummings J, et al. Pulmonary-vein isolation for atrial fibrillation in patients with heart failure. N Engl J Med 2008;359(17):1778–85.

51. Wann LS, Curtis AB, January CT, et al. 2011 ACCF/AHA/HRS focused update on the management of patients with atrial fibrillation (Updating the 2006 Guideline): a report of the American College of Cardiology Foundation/American Heart Association Task Force on Practice Guidelines. J Am Coll Cardiol 2011;57(2):223–42.

52. Deedwania PC, Lardizabal JA. Non-antiarrhythmic therapies. In: Saksena S, John C, editors. Electrophysiological disorders of the heart. 2nd edition. Oxford (UK): Churchill-Livingstone; 2011. p. 82–3.

53. Zhang L, Zhang S, Jiang H, et al. Effects of statin treatment on cardiac function in patients with chronic heart failure: a meta-analysis of randomized controlled trials. Clin Cardiol 2011;34(2):117–23.

54. Nodari S, Triggiani M, Campia U, et al. Effects of n-3 polyunsaturated fatty acids on left ventricular function and functional capacity in patients with dilated cardiomyopathy. J Am Coll Cardiol 2011;57(7):870–9.

55. Rastogi S, Sharov VG, Mishra S, et al. Ranolazine combined with enalapril or metoprolol prevents progressive LV dysfunction and remodeling in dogs with moderate heart failure. Am J Physiol Heart Circ Physiol 2008;295(5):H2149–55.

56. Schneider MP, Hua TA, Böhm M, et al. Prevention of atrial fibrillation by Renin-Angiotensin system inhibition a meta-analysis. J Am Coll Cardiol 2010;55(21):2299–307.

57. ACTIVE-I Investigators. Irbesartan in patients with atrial fibrillation. N Engl J Med 2011;364(10):928–38.

58. Shammas FV, Dickstein K. Clinical pharmacokinetics in heart failure: an updated review. Clin Pharmacokinet 1988;15(2):94–113.

59. Connolly SJ, Ezekowitz MD, Yusuf S, et al. Dabigatran versus warfarin in patients with atrial fibrillation. N Engl J Med 2009;361(12):1139–51.

60. Wann LS, Curtis AB, Ellenbogen KA, et al. 2011 ACCF/AHA/HRS Focused Update on the Management of Patients With Atrial Fibrillation (Update on Dabigatran). A Report of the American College of Cardiology Foundation Foundation/American Heart Association Task Force on Practice Guidelines. J Am Coll Cardiol 2011;57(11):1330–7.

61. Connolly S, Pogue J, Hart R, et al. Clopidogrel plus aspirin versus oral anticoagulation for atrial fibrillation in the Atrial fibrillation Clopidogrel Trial with Irbesartan for prevention of Vascular Events (ACTIVE W): a randomised controlled trial. Lancet 2006;367(9526):1903–12.

Breast Cancer Therapies and Cardiomyopathy

John Groarke, MBBChBAO, MSc[a], Dan Tong, MD, PhD[a],
Jay Khambhati, BA, BS[a], Susan Cheng, MD[a], Javid Moslehi, MD[a,b,*]

KEYWORDS

- Breast cancer • Cardiomyopathy • Transthoracic echocardiography
- Multi-gated radionuclide angiography

KEY POINTS

- The prevalence of chemotherapy-related cardiac disease is increasing and management requires a multidisciplinary approach from cardiologists and oncologists.
- Pretreatment identification of predisposing risk factors and assessment of cardiac function before and at intervals during and after therapy with cardiotoxic agents are necessary.
- In clinical practice, surveillance is largely performed using transthoracic echocardiography or multi-gated radionuclide angiography. Imaging strategies that detect cardiac injury before overt left ventricular systolic dysfunction provide an opportunity for early intervention and improved cardiac outcomes.

 Video 1: Non-dilated, globally hypokinetic left ventricle and mild dilatation of the right ventricle. Video 2: Normal left ventricular function available at http://www. medical.theclinics.com/

CASE VIGNETTE

A 41-year-old woman with no previous cardiac history was diagnosed with stage II invasive ductal carcinoma of the right breast. Pathology confirmed that the tumor was estrogen receptor negative, progesterone receptor negative, and human epidermal receptor (HER)-2 positive. Initial chemotherapy consisted of doxorubicin, to a cumulative dose of 240 mg/m^2, and adjuvant cyclophosphamide. Transthoracic echocardiography on completion of this regimen revealed left ventricular systolic dysfunction, with an estimated left ventricular ejection fraction (LVEF) of 40% to

[a] Division of Cardiovascular Medicine, Department of Medicine, Brigham and Women's Hospital, 75 Francis Street, Boston, MA 02115, USA; [b] Division of Medical Oncology, Early Drug Development Center, Lance Armstrong Foundation, Dana-Farber Cancer Institute, Harvard Medical School, 450 Brookline Avenue, Boston, MA 02115, USA
* Corresponding author. Cardio-Oncology Program, Brigham and Women's Hospital, Dana-Farber Cancer Institute, 75 Francis Street, Boston, MA 02115.
E-mail address: jmoslehi@partners.org

Med Clin N Am 96 (2012) 1001–1019
http://dx.doi.org/10.1016/j.mcna.2012.07.008
0025-7125/12/$ – see front matter © 2012 Published by Elsevier Inc.

medical.theclinics.com

45% (Video 1), whereas pretreatment LVEF had been normal at 60%. Her oncologist had planned to commence adjuvant trastuzumab, a monoclonal antibody targeting HER2, because a meta-analysis of randomized controlled trials suggested that adjuvant trastuzumab would offer this patient a 34% lower relative risk of mortality, a 36% lower relative risk of locoregional recurrence, and 40% lower relative risk of distant recurrence compared with chemotherapy without trastuzumab.[1] She was referred to the cardio-oncology clinic for further evaluation and management of her cardiomyopathy and for assessment of cardiac suitability for trastuzumab therapy.

INTRODUCTION

The advent of modern cancer therapy has considerably improved the outcomes of oncology patients and, for the first time, has introduced *survivorship* as a theme in the management of patients with cancer. However, both traditional and novel chemotherapies are associated with cardiotoxicity. Increasingly, patients with cancer are older, have cardiovascular comorbidities, have prior exposure to anticancer therapies, and/or have received combinations of agents. These factors can predispose to cardiotoxic effects of chemotherapies and contribute to a growing prevalence of patients with cardiac diseases related to cancer treatments. Cardio-oncology services are emerging internationally to guide optimal management of this challenging patient population.

The more common anticancer therapies and their respective cardiotoxicities are outlined in **Table 1**. This review focuses on cardiomyopathy associated with anthracycline chemotherapies and HER-2 targeted therapies, which together constitute a major subset of referrals to cardio-oncology clinics. Cardiomyopathy in the setting of these agents can range from asymptomatic reversible myocardial injury to irreversible, symptomatic congestive heart failure. Surveillance and management strategies used to identify and treat adverse cardiac effects for these chemotherapies are reviewed. The challenges facing cardio-oncologists are also explored, including the lack of consensus guidelines to direct clinical practice.

ANTHRACYCLINE-INDUCED CARDIOMYOPATHY

Anthracyclines serve as effective chemotherapy for the treatment of breast cancer, acute leukemia, Hodgkin and non-Hodgkin lymphoma, and sarcomas—all of which are cancer types that can occur in young people and are potentially curable. Doxorubicin (Adriamycin) and daunorubicin (daunomycin) are glycoside antibiotics and were the original anthracyclines isolated from the pigment-producing bacterium *Streptomyces peucetius* in the 1960s. The precise mechanisms of action of anthracyclines are still debated but likely involve tumor DNA intercalation, DNA binding and alkylation, increased DNA damage via the generation of reactive oxygen species, inhibition of topoisomerase II, and induction of apoptosis. Anthracyclines, and specifically doxorubicin, remain an important cornerstone of chemotherapy for a vast variety of cancers and are increasingly being used in older patient populations.

In initial trials with doxorubicin and daunorubicin, toxicities were noted in tissues with a high mitotic rate, such as the bone marrow, gastrointestinal system, and hair follicles. Accordingly, many patients suffered from nausea, vomiting, myelosuppression, and alopecia[2]; but these toxicities were generally reversible or responsive to drug dose adjustments. It later came as a surprise when further studies with doxorubicin indicated that the major limitation of use was cardiac toxicity. Clinicians now widely recognize that anthracyclines pose a significant cardiac risk, which can manifest as a reversible early (or acute) cardiac toxicity and/or a later (chronic) presentation of cardiomyopathy with

Table 1
Commonly prescribed anticancer agents with summary of respective cardiotoxicity profiles

Class	Commonly Prescribed Agents	Trade Name	Incidence of Cardiotoxicity[a] (%) (Incidence of Left Ventricular Dysfuntion -%)	Reversibility
Anthracyclines	Doxorubicin Epirubicin	Adriamycin Ellence	Dose dependent; up to 26[b]	+
HER-2 targeted therapies				
A. Monoclonal Antibodies	Trastuzumab	Herceptin	4.5[c] (up to 30% with asymptomatic cardiomyopathy)	+++
B. TKIs	Lapatinib	Tykerb	1.5–2.2[g]	Uncertain
VSP inhibitors				
A. Monoclonal Antibodies	Bevacizumab	Avastin	2.2[h]	Uncertain
B. TKIs	Sorafenib Sunitinib	Nexavar Sutent	2.1[d] 4.1[e]	+++
Other Tyrosine Kinase Inhibitors (TKIs)	Imatinib	Gleevec	1.7[f]	Uncertain

Abbreviations: HER2, human epidermal growth factor receptor 2; TKI, tyrosine kinase inhibitor; VSP, vascular endothelial growth factor signaling pathway.

[a] Note: Definitions of cardiotoxicity used by sources vary, limiting direct comparisons of incidence between agents. Reversibility indicates the percentage of patients who have cardiomyopathy reversibility after cessation of drug treatment and/or initiation of cardioprotective medications. "+" denotes least likely to reverse and "++++" most reversible. We additionally suggest changing the class grades as follow: anthracyclines "+", Her-2 receptor targeted therapies "+++" and TKIs under VSP inhibitors (see below for clarification of table 1) "+++".

[b] Jensen. Semin Oncol. 2006;33:S15–21.

[c] Suter, Procter M, van Veldhuisen DJ, et al. J Clin Oncol. 2007:25:3859–65.

[d] Escudier, Eisen T, Stadler WM, et al. N Engl J Med. 2007;356(2):125.

[e] Richards, Je Y, Schutz FA, et al. J Clin Oncol. 2011;29(25):3450.

[f] Atallah, Durand JB, Kantarjian H, et al. Blood. 2007;110(4):1233.

[g] Perez, Koehler M, Byrne J, et al. Mayo Clin Proc. 2008;83(6):679.

[h] Brana Choueiri TK, Mayer EL, Je Y, et al. J Clin Oncol. 2011;29(6):632–8.

clinical heart failure and associated mortality. More recently, it has become evident that myocardial injury can occur at the time of acute treatment with doxorubicin and that, conversely, doxorubicin-induced chronic cardiomyopathy is potentially reversible.

Acute Cardiotoxicity

Acutely, anthracycline treatment can cause tachycardia, hypotension, electrocardiographic changes, arrhythmias, and a myocarditis-pericarditis syndrome. In rare cases, myocardial infarction or even sudden cardiac death can occur within hours following anthracycline treatment. Nonetheless, *acute* cardiovascular complications are largely asymptomatic and are generally thought to be reversible.[3] In a study of almost 1700 patients with non-Hodgkin lymphoma, 55 patients developed acute cardiotoxicity requiring a cardiology referral, including 5 cases of acute heart failure and 1 case of myocardial infarction.[4] Older patients, who are more likely to have coexisting cardiovascular disease, seem to be predisposed to the acute cardiotoxicities associated with doxorubicin.[5] In a study evaluating the use of liposomal doxorubicin in an older patient cohort (mean age of 72 years), 1 out of every 5 patients developed acute cardiotoxicity, including tachycardia, atrial fibrillation, and cardiomyopathy.[6]

Although acute cardiotoxicity associated with anthracyclines has been traditionally thought to be reversible, recent studies have highlighted the potential for irreversible myocardial injury. At the time of infusion-based administration of anthracyclines, elevation of serum troponins have been detected.[7] Furthermore, myocardial biopsies obtained within hours after anthracycline exposure have demonstrated evidence of myocardial tissue injury and cell death.[8] Evidence of anthracycline-induced myocyte damage has also been seen in children in whom troponin elevations have been correlated with later left ventricular remodeling on echocardiography.[9] More studies are needed to determine whether acute cardiotoxicity after anthracycline exposure predicts future cardiomyopathy or heart failure.

Chronic Cardiotoxicity

Chronic cardiovascular toxicities associated with anthracyclines are a cause for even greater concern. Cardiomyopathy and clinical heart failure are the main dose-limiting side effects of anthracyclines. Anthracycline-induced cardiomyopathy can occur within the first year and up to a decade after completion of therapy. A recent meta-analysis showed that the use of an anthracycline-based chemotherapy was associated with a significant increased risk of both clinical and subclinical cardiotoxicity over use of a non-anthracycline-based chemotherapy.[10] Initial studies suggested an incidence of 2.2% of developing clinical congestive heart failure after doxorubicin treatment.[11] A significantly higher percentage of patients have evidence of subclinical heart failure. Fifty-seven percent of children exposed to doxorubicin had echocardiographic evidence of cardiac dysfunction, although only 10% had clinical heart failure.[12] In a separate study of adult survivors of childhood cancer, most of whom were treated with anthracyclines, 27% of the patients had echocardiographic evidence of cardiac dysfunction.[13]

Several risk factors predispose patients to anthracycline-induced cardiomyopathy. The strongest predictor for cardiac dysfunction is the cumulative dose of anthracyclines administered.[14] In the case of doxorubicin, general recommendations dictate the cumulative dose of doxorubicin not to exceed 450 mg/m^2 in adults. However, there is variability seen among patients, with some developing heart failure at a cumulative dose of 300 mg/m^2. Other risk factors predisposing to anthracyclines-induced cardiomyopathy include age extremes, concomitant chemotherapy and radiation, and a history of cardiovascular disease. Although preexisting cardiac history or cardiac risk factors may potentiate the development of doxorubicin-induced heart failure in older patients, it is less clear why children are at an increased risk of developing anthracycline-induced cardiomyopathy, where a younger age is associated with echocardiographic evidence of cardiac dysfunction.[15]

Pathogenesis

Most proposed models for anthracycline-induced cardiomyopathy suggest progressive myocardial cell death following successive anthracycline exposure.[16] Although earlier stages of anthracycline-induced cardiac damage may be undetectable via standard cardiac imaging, cumulative exposure to anthracyclines eventually exceeds a threshold of myocardial damage that manifests initially as overt structural cardiac changes (eg, myocardial dilatation, cardiomyopathy) and ultimately as frank heart failure. Acute exposure to anthracyclines leads to myocardial damage, as evidenced by elevated cardiac serum biomarkers and histologic changes on myocardial biopsy, including mitochondrial swelling and chromatin contraction, consistent with apoptosis.[16]

Less clear are the upstream pathways leading to myocardial cell death. The presumed mechanism of action of anthracyclines is interference with DNA replication in rapidly dividing cells, such as cancer cells. Consistent with this hypothesis, some side effects of anthracyclines are seen in organs with high turnover, such as bone marrow and hair follicles. It is, therefore, surprising that the heart (an organ with limited regenerative capacity) is the major organ of toxicity. The proposed mechanism of cardiotoxicity is the generation of reactive oxygen species by various mechanisms including redox cycling, iron complexation, and electron transport chain uncoupling. Accordingly, overexpression of free of radical scavengers, or co-treatment with strong antioxidants, protects against anthracyclines-induced cardiomyopathy in animal models. However, these preclinical studies have not translated to human clinical trials, indicating that oxidative stress may not be the sole mechanism of toxicity.[17]

Aside from standard cardioprotective medications, the only compound that has been found to be consistently protective in anthracycline-mediated cardiomyopathy has been dexrazoxane, an iron chelator that can attenuate iron-catalyzed hydroxyl radical formation. Dexrazoxane prevents or reduces cardiac injury, as reflected by elevations in troponin T and long-term echocardiographic measures of cardiac remodeling in children treated with leukemia.[18,19] More studies are needed to assess clinical end points such as incident heart failure or cardiac death. Notably, the use of dexrazoxane has met some resistance in the adult oncology community due to a perceived risk of secondary malignant formation.

HER2 TARGETED THERAPY

The human epidermal growth factor receptors (EGF receptors or ErbB) are a family of transmembrane receptor tyrosine kinases involved in the regulation of cell growth and cell survival, with important roles in tumor genesis and growth.[20,21] HER2, one of the 4 members of this family, is overexpressed in about 20% to 30% of breast cancers and is often associated with a more aggressive tumor phenotype associated with a poorer prognosis.[22–25] HER2 overexpression in cancer cells leads to continuous stimulation of downstream signaling pathways and uncontrolled cell proliferation.[26]

Trastuzumab (Herceptin), a humanized monoclonal antibody against the extracellular domain of the HER2 protein that can inhibit proliferation of malignant cells, is approved for the treatment of both metastatic and early stage breast cancer with HER2 overexpression.[22] A meta-analysis of 5 randomized controlled trials comparing chemotherapy with and without trastuzumab in 13 493 women with HER2-positive breast cancer reported a 34% lower relative risk of mortality, a 36% lower relative risk of locoregional recurrence, and a 40% lower relative risk of distant recurrence among patients receiving trastuzumab.[1] Lapatinib is another Food and Drug Administration–approved second-line agent for use with capecitabine for HER2-positive metastatic breast cancer, or for use in combination with letrozole for hormone receptor–positive disease.[27] Unlike trastuzumab, lapatinib is an oral small tyrosine kinase inhibitor (TKI) that competes with ATP for binding to the ATP binding pocket of kinases HER1 and HER2, blocking phosphorylation and activation of both receptors.[28] Phase III trials showed that adjuvant lapatinib improves outcomes in patients with advanced breast cancer overexpressing HER2.[29,30] More recently, pertuzumab, a monoclonal antibody that inhibits HER2 dimerization and activation, as well as the antibody-drug composite, trastuzumab emtansine (also known as T-DM1), have shown efficacy in patients with HER2-positive breast cancer. These novel therapies illustrate an expanding arsenal of HER2-targeted therapies that are being used, often in combination, for HER2-positive breast cancer.

Cardiotoxicity

Trastuzumab can cause an asymptomatic decline in cardiac function as well as symptomatic congestive heart failure. In early clinical trials, trastuzumab was given concomitantly with other chemotherapies for breast cancer treatment, resulting in a variable incidence of heart failure. For example, patients treated with trastuzumab and along with concurrent anthracycline and cyclophosphamide had an incidence of symptomatic cardiac dysfunction of 27%, with the incidence decreasing to 13% in the setting of paclitaxel and trastuzumab combination therapy.[22] In subsequent trials, trastuzumab was given sequentially following other chemotherapies, resulting in a significant decrease in the incidence of cardiomyopathy. In these studies, the incidence of severe symptomatic (New York Heart Association class III or IV) heart failure in patients treated with chemotherapy and adjuvant trastuzumab was found to range from 0.5% to 3.7% compared with 0% up to 0.7% among patients treated with chemotherapy alone.[1] The incidence of asymptomatic reductions in LVEF was higher and resulted in the discontinuation of trastuzumab in approximately 14% of patients in one study.[31] In contrast, in a pooled analysis of 44 clinical trials, only 1.6% of 3689 patients treated with lapatinib experienced a 20% or more decrease in LVEF relative to baseline and most were asymptomatic.[32]

Cardiac dysfunction caused by trastuzumab differs from anthracycline-induced cardiomyopathy in that it is not dose dependent; it can occur acutely, even after the first exposure; and, it is largely reversible on treatment withdrawal. These differences have led to the subclassification of chemotherapy-associated cardiomyopathies into type I (anthracycline-like, which presumably involves myocyte death) and type II cardiomyopathy (trastuzumab-like, where there is reversibility of myocardial impairment).[33] These subtypes are not mutually exclusive and may coexist in patients treated with contemporary multi-agent treatment regimens.

Pathophysiology

The pathophysiological mechanisms underlying trastuzumab-induced cardiotoxicity are not fully understood. The activation of HER2/HER4 heterodimers by neuregulin1 (NRG1), a growth factor produced by cardiac endothelial cells, stimulates many important downstream signaling pathways that promote cardiomyocyte growth and survival.[34–37] By specifically blocking HER2, trastuzumab treatment appears to compromise the ability of myocytes to withstand or recover from stressors, such as anthracycline-induced damage. Mitochondrial dysfunction and disruption of ATP production have also been postulated as a possible mechanism for trastuzumab-associated cardiotoxicity.[38,39] The relatively lower incidence of cardiotoxicity observed with lapatinib, which also blocks the NRG/ErbB pathway, is puzzling. A few hypotheses have been proposed. As a monoclonal antibody, trastuzumab may mediate antibody-dependent cell cytotoxicity and complement-dependent cytotoxicity, thus augmenting cardiotoxicity.[28,40] Furthermore, differential inhibition or activation of downstream signaling pathways by lapatinib versus trastuzumab may also explain observed discrepancies in outcomes.[41]

DIAGNOSIS

Maintaining an index of suspicion for cardiotoxicity in patients receiving cancer therapies is fundamental for timely diagnosis. A review of symptoms and clinical examination at regular intervals before, during, and after chemotherapy are necessary. However, cardiotoxicity is often subclinical until a certain threshold of injury is exceeded, limiting the sensitivity of symptoms and signs of heart failure in early diagnosis of cardiac injury. Therefore, cardiac imaging and cardiac biomarkers are complementary in the diagnosis and screening of patients with possible chemotherapy-induced cardiotoxicity.

Cardiac Imaging

Transthoracic echocardiography

In current clinical practice, transthoracic echocardiography (TTE) and multi-gated radionuclide angiography (MUGA) are the most commonly used modalities for non-invasive baseline and serial assessment of LVEF in patients receiving chemotherapeutic agents. TTE provides a qualitative and quantitative assessment of LVEF, in addition to useful information regarding valvular function, pericardial processes, and diastolic function. It should be noted that TTE image quality and interpretation can be limited in patients with obesity, chronic obstructive pulmonary disease, and musculoskeletal deformities. For such cases, contrast-enhanced echocardiography can improve endocardial definition allowing for accurate and reproducible assessments of LVEF.[42,43] The diagnosis of cardiotoxicity relies on the detection of often subtle differences in LVEF, underscoring the need for echocardiogram reports to detail any quality issues that might compromise the reliability of results.

MUGA

MUGA assessments of LV systolic and diastolic function are commonly used. MUGA provides a well-established, simple, reproducible, and accurate measurement of LV function. Oncologists' familiarity with this technique and interpreting results likely contribute to the pervasive presence of MUGA in contemporary surveillance strategies. Unlike TTE, MUGA exposes patients to radiation and fails to provide additional information on valvular and pericardial processes, which are not infrequent complications of cancer and cancer therapies. Surveillance schedules have been suggested for monitoring patients with serial MUGAs for doxorubicin-induced cardiotoxicity; monitoring LVEF in accordance with these protocols has been associated with a fourfold reduction in the incidence of doxorubicin-associated heart failure.[44]

Novel imaging techniques

Echocardiography: myocardial strain and tissue Doppler imaging Deterioration in LV systolic function to the point that it is manifest as a noticeable change in LVEF is a relatively late and potentially irreversible finding. More sensitive imaging strategies that may identify cardiotoxicity at an earlier, modifiable stage in the disease process are under review. Interest has focused particularly on the contemporary echocardiographic techniques of tissue Doppler and myocardial strain imaging.

Reductions in LV diastolic function may precede LV systolic function in chemotherapy-induced cardiotoxicity (**Fig. 1**).[45,46] Several small and largely single-center studies have reported observing utility in assessing serial changes in radionuclide angiography or TTE-derived measurements of LV diastolic function in the effort to detect subclinical cardiotoxicity.[1,2,47,48] However, serial echocardiographic assessment of diastolic parameters failed to predict cardiotoxicity among 43 patients receiving anthracycline and trastuzumab as the treatment of breast cancer.[49] Such small, single-center studies with inconsistent findings highlight the need for larger multicenter prospective studies to determine the role for serial quantification of diastolic function.

Longitudinal myocardial strain echocardiography has also been reported in several small studies as more sensitive than conventional LVEF assessment in the early detection of LV cardiotoxicity (**Fig. 2**).[50,51] An early decrease (>10%) in peak systolic myocardial longitudinal strain predicted the later occurrence of cardiotoxicity among 43 patients receiving anthracyclines and trastuzumab with a sensitivity and specificity of 78% and 79%, respectively.[49] Among 81 women treated with anthracyclines followed by taxanes and trastuzumab, abnormalities of peak systolic longitudinal myocardial strain measured after completion of anthracycline therapy predicted

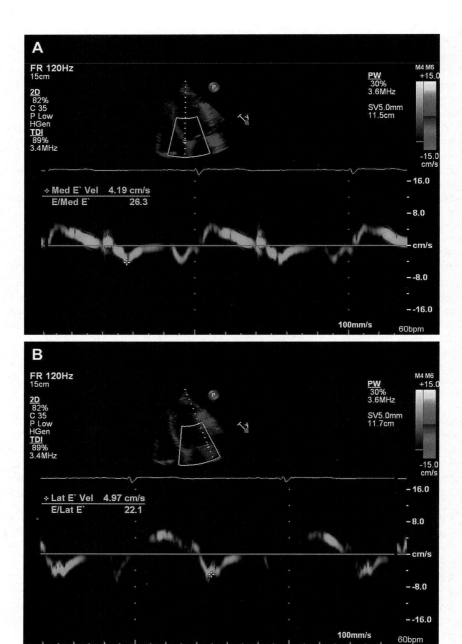

Fig. 1. (*A*) Pulsed-wave (PW) analysis of mitral annular velocity at the septal wall is obtained with tissue Doppler imaging (TDI). Med E′ Vel (medial early myocardial velocity) of 4.19 cm/s is lower than the reference range of normal (12.2 ± 2.3 cm/s) for this 46-year-old female patient with preserved LVEF receiving doxorubicin. (*B*) PW of the mitral annulus (lateral wall) obtained by TDI from the same patient. Lat E′ Vel (lateral early myocardial velocity) of 4.97 cm/s is also lower than the reference range of normal for this patient (16.1 ± 2.3 cm/s). These findings confirm the presence of impaired left ventricular relaxation (diastolic dysfunction), which may be an earlier marker of cardiotoxicity compared to overt changes in LV systolic function.

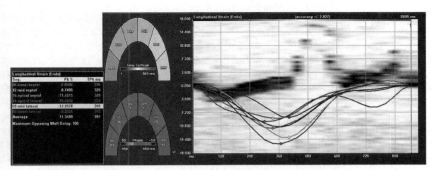

Fig. 2. Longitudinal strain analysis performed on the apical 4-chamber view. The 7 curves represent longitudinal myocardial strain (*y* axis) over a single cardiac cycle (*x* axis) for each of 6 LV segments (basal septum [*green*], midseptal [*white*], apical septal [*light blue*], apical lateral [*dark blue*], midlateral [*yellow*], basal lateral [*pink*]) and a gray curve that represents the average (global) longitudinal strain of these 6 segments. The numerical values for peak longitudinal strain for each of these segments are outlined in the adjacent table. In a study of 240 healthy volunteers, mean (±SD) overall global longitudinal strain was −18.6 ± 5.1%. The strain analysis in this figure was performed on a 46-year-old woman with normal LVEF who recently completed anthracycline chemotherapy; a mean peak systolic longitudinal myocardial strain of −11.4% is abnormal and is associated with increased risk of subsequent cardiomyopathy, indicating the need for surveillance assessment of LVEF. (*Data from* Marwick TH, Leano RL, Brown J, et al. Myocardial Strain Measurement With 2-Dimensional Speckle-Tracking Echocardiography. J Am Coll Cardiol Img 2009;2:80–4.)

subsequent cardiotoxicity.[7] Eighteen (51%) out of 35 patients undergoing trastuzumab therapy for breast cancer demonstrated significant reductions in longitudinal strain, identifying preclinical myocardial dysfunction before standard echocardiographic measures, such as LVEF.[52]

Serial real-time 3-dimensional TTE (RT3DTTE) assessment of LV end-diastolic volumes (LVEDVs) has been shown to strongly correlate with measurements of cardiac magnetic resonance imaging (CMR) and/or MUGA-derived measurements of LVEDV in a cohort of 50 female patients with breast cancer who received trastuzumab after doxorubicin.[53] As imaging technology advances and experience with acquisition and post-processing accumulates, RT3DTE may assume an important role as a reliable and reproducible alternative to 2-dimensional TTE assessment of LV volumes. The additive value of dobutamine or exercise stress echocardiography in the early detection and surveillance of cardiotoxicity is uncertain, with inconsistent results from small single-center studies.[54–56]

Nuclear imaging techniques Nuclear imaging techniques that detect myocardial injury at an early stage preceding the development of overt LV systolic dysfunction are under investigation. Such techniques include ^{123}I-labeled meta-iodobenzylguanidine (MIBG) scintigraphy (decreased ^{123}I-MIBG uptake in cases of doxorubicin-induced cardiomyopathy), cardiac sympathetic neuronal imaging using positron-emission tomography (PET), and ^{111}In-antimyosin scintigraphy (^{111}In-antimyosin binds to intracellular myosin of injured myocytes).[57] It will be necessary to standardize acquisition protocols and to clarify the role and utility of these techniques through clinical studies before their application in practice.

CMR CMR allows very accurate and reproducible assessment of ventricular volumes and estimation of LVEF. T2-weighted imaging with fat suppression can detect myocardial edema that may be a feature of acute myocardial inflammation and injury secondary to carditoxicity[58]; the role of this technique in the diagnosis of cardiotoxicity and the clinical significance of myocardial edema in this context requires evaluation in prospective studies. The pattern and significance of late gadolinium enhancement (LGE) in patients with cardiotoxicity also requires investigation. Subepicardial linear LGE of the lateral segments of the LV has been described in patients with trastuzumab-induced cardiomyopathy.[59] Relatively limited access, cost, and time required for acquisition and post-processing limit the practical use of CMR technology in routine surveillance for cardiotoxicity. However, CMR may be more practically employed in the single-use evaluation of patients with manifest LV dysfunction following exposure to chemotherapy. In such patients, CMR can assist in evaluating for alternative or contributing disease processes such as ischemic heart disease and infiltrative disorders.

Appropriate use criteria

Concerns about potential overutilization of various cardiac imaging modalities led to the development of appropriate use criteria for each modality by the various academic bodies, such as the American College of Cardiology and American Heart Association. The use of TTE or MUGA is considered appropriate in the baseline and serial evaluation of patients undergoing therapy with cardiotoxic agents.[60,61] CMR is considered appropriate in the evaluation of LV function in patients with technically challenging echocardiograms and/or in the evaluation of cardiomyopathies caused by cardiotoxic therapies.[62]

Cardiac Biomarkers

Elevated troponin or NT-pro-brain natriuretic peptide (BNP) in the early post-exposure period can identify an at-risk subgroup that may benefit from increased frequency of cardiac function testing.[7,63–66] Elevated ultrasensitive troponin I assays exceeding 30 pg/mL at the completion of anthracycline therapy were predictive of subsequent cardiotoxicity in a study of 81 patients with breast cancer.[7] Persistently elevated NT-pro-BNP assays in the early aftermath of high-dose chemotherapy were strongly associated with downstream cardiac dysfunction among 52 patients treated with high-dose chemotherapy.[66] In clinical practice, it is likely that the utility of biomarkers will prove most helpful as an adjunct to cardiac imaging in the intensified surveillance of patients predisposed to cardiotoxicity for the detection of earlier subclinical toxicity, directing more timely interventions and surveillance schedules.

MANAGEMENT

The management of chemotherapy-induced cardiomyopathy requires a multidisciplinary approach with input from both the oncology and cardiology teams. Benefits of continuing chemotherapy and/or modifying treatment regimens must be weighed against the risk of irreversible cardiovascular outcomes. The development of cardiooncology programs will help to deliver experience and expertise in the management of this growing and challenging patient population.

Surveillance

Cardiac imaging–based surveillance of LV function during treatment with agents other than trastuzumab remains controversial. In the case of trastuzumab, the timing of surveillance cardiac function tests generally adheres to pretreatment baseline studies and then quarterly studies for the duration of chemotherapy.[49,67,68] The frequency of studies following the completion of chemotherapy varies without consensus. The protocol followed in the authors' institution for patients receiving trastuzumab is outlined in **Fig. 3**.

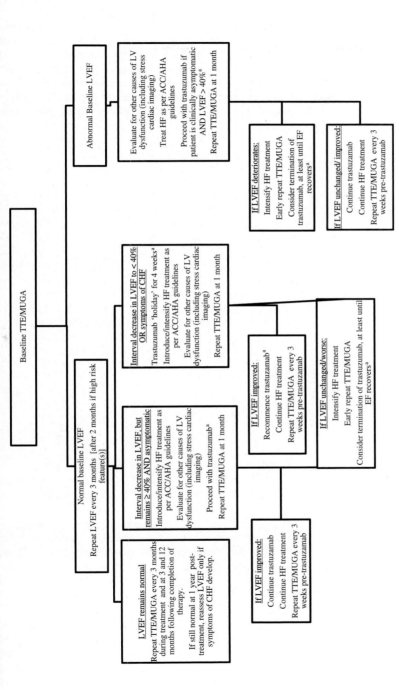

Fig. 3. Local institutional algorithm for cardiac surveillance of patients receiving trastuzumab with or without prior exposure to chemotherapy. [a] Requires consensus of cardiologist and oncologist following risk-benefit analysis. ACC, American College of Cardiology; AHA, American Heart Association; HF, Heart Failure; EF, Ejection Fraction.

There are currently no published consensus guidelines on the prospective surveillance and management of cardiotoxic effects of cancer therapies in adults.[69]

The concept of a standard surveillance schedule is arbitrary. Individual susceptibility to cardiotoxicity and the cardiotoxic potential of all anticancer treatments are not uniform. Thus, a reasonable approach is to tailor surveillance schedules according to patient susceptibility and the agent involved. Patients require pretreatment screening for characteristics associated with increased risk of cardiotoxicity. Identifying high-risk patients should prompt intensified surveillance of cardiac function.[70] High-risk features that are largely relevant in the context of exposure to any potentially cardiotoxic drug treatment are outlined in **Box 1**.

Pharmacotherapy

In the context of established LV systolic impairment that is presumed secondary to anti-cancer therapy, heart failure therapies, including beta-blockers and angiotensin converting enzyme (ACE) inhibitors or angiotensin receptor blockers, are introduced and up-titrated according to contemporary guidelines for the management of heart failure.[71] Studies of heart failure treatments specifically in patients with chemotherapy-induced cardiomyopathy are few. The addition of enalapril, with or without carvedilol, was studied in a single-center prospective study of 201 patients with anthracycline-induced cardiomyopathy (LVEF $\leq$45%), and was associated with some improvement in LV function in 55% of patients.[72] In the absence of specific guidelines, standard pharmacotherapy of heart failure should also be initiated in the setting of trastuzumab-induced cardiomyopathy. Given the preclinical and clinical evidence in favor of dexrazoxane, prophylactic use should be considered in high-risk patients being treated with anthracyclines. The optimal heart failure regimen for chemotherapy-induced cardiotoxicity requires evaluation through dedicated clinical trials.

Balancing Cancer and Cardiovascular Outcomes

The main challenge of cardio-oncology is to balance cancer and cardiovascular outcomes. An overall aim is to avoid compromising the efficacy of anti-cancer therapy while minimizing the risk of cardiac side effects. The evidence base to achieve such goals is deficient and consensus is lacking. This deficiency emphasizes the need to include cardiac outcomes in the design of trials for anti-cancer therapies, extend follow-up periods to detect late cardiotoxicity, and determine optimal cost-effective surveillance strategies and schedules for the early detection of cardiotoxicity. The clinical significance of abnormalities in ventricular strain and diastolic measurements, myocardial edema on

---

Box 1
General risk factors that predispose to cardiotoxic effects of anti-cancer drugs

Very young (applies to anthracyclines) or old age at exposure

Combination of anti-cancer agents

Prior exposure to anti-cancer agents

Radiation therapy that included the heart or part of the heart in the irradiated volume

Cumulative dose (applies to anthracyclines)

Baseline LV dysfunction

Cardiovascular risk factors (eg, hypertension, diabetes mellitus)

Elevated troponin and/or NT-pro-BNP assays early following exposure

T2-weighted magnetic resonance imaging, and abnormalities on nuclear functional imaging need to be evaluated by prospective trials. Overinterpreting the clinical significance of such findings may prompt modifications to anti-cancer therapies at the cost of efficacy. On the other hand, such findings may present an opportunity for early intervention that may reduce the risk of downstream, irreversible cardiac morbidity.

Recommendations

There are certain key concepts that are clinically applied at the authors' institution. All patients undergoing therapy with a potentially cardiotoxic agent require a baseline pretreatment study of cardiac function. Although the need is apparent, cardiac testing pretreatment is underutilized. For example, less than 30% of 3779 women with metastatic breast cancer receiving trastuzumab between 2001 and 2010 had pretreatment cardiac function testing.[73] The authors encourage pretreatment screening of all patients for the high-risk features outlined in **Box 1** and advocate surveillance for specific high-risk cohorts. Serial TTE with the measurement of LV systolic and diastolic parameters, in addition to myocardial strain and strain rate imaging, and direct comparison with equivalent measures on prior studies is the contemporary default surveillance strategy in the authors' institution, maintaining a low threshold for using ultrasound contrast agents as needed.

It is important to remember that LVEF measured by the differing modalities of MUGA, TTE, and CMR are not interchangeable.[74] Therefore, the same modality is used throughout surveillance for reliable interval comparisons.

For patients with established LV systolic dysfunction, additional cardiac testing is considered on an individual patient basis. Stress imaging can help exclude ischemia as an alternative cause of or contributor to LV impairment. Several stress-imaging modalities are useful in this context and selection will be governed by local availability and expertise. Stress CMR offers the advantage of evaluating for ischemia while also providing useful additional information, including accurate quantification of LV volumes and information on the pattern of any myocardial edema or LGE that may be present. However, patients with contraindications to magnetic resonance imaging (MRI) (eg, pacemaker) or significant renal dysfunction precluding administration of gadolinium are not suitable for this technique. Stress myocardial perfusion imaging with single-photon emission computed tomography or PET-computed tomography (CT) are alternatives for evaluating for ischemia; PET-CT offers the advantages of lower radiation exposure and the ability to quantify coronary flow reserve.

SUMMARY

The pharmacologic armamentarium used in the treatment of all stages of cancer has evolved in recent decades, and ongoing oncology clinical trials promise further progress. As such, drug regimens used in the treatment of cancer are increasingly complex with combinations of agents with differing, and sometimes synergistic, cardiotoxic potential.

Clinical trials of chemotherapeutic approaches have been criticized for inconsistent definitions of cardiotoxicity, variable cardiac surveillance strategies and schedules, and failure to monitor diastolic function.[75] Furthermore, trials may fail to include cardiac endpoints in the study design, and follow-up durations are often insufficient to detect late cardiotoxicity. These factors contribute to uncertainty of the true incidence of cardiotoxicity for many anticancer agents. The prevalence of chemotherapy-related cardiac disease is increasing and management demands a multidisciplinary approach from cardiologists and oncologists.

Pretreatment identification of predisposing risk factors and the assessment of cardiac function before and at intervals during and after therapy with cardiotoxic agents are necessary. In clinical practice, surveillance is largely performed using TTE or MUGA. Imaging strategies that detect cardiac injury before overt LV systolic dysfunction provide an opportunity for early intervention and improved cardiac outcomes. Appropriately designed clinical trials are needed to clarify optimal surveillance strategies and schedules, the cost-effectiveness of various approaches, and the appropriate management based on imaging findings.

EPILOGUE

The patient presented in the case vignette was immediately initiated on an ACE inhibitor and a beta-blocker, with up-titration of each to the maximum tolerated doses. Cardiovascular risk factor screening did not identify any additional contributing or alternative cause for cardiomyopathy. Cardiac MRI was negative for stress-induced perfusion abnormalities, demonstrating a nonspecific, nondilated cardiomyopathy with an LVEF of 41%. A diagnosis of anthracycline-associated cardiomyopathy was made.

Repeat TTE performed 4 weeks after the initiation of heart failure therapy confirmed an interval improvement in LVEF from 45% to 50%. Given the compelling survival advantage offered by trastuzumab for the patient's cancer type, the multidisciplinary consensus was to commence trastuzumab and continue heart failure therapies concurrently.

Surveillance TTE was performed every 3 weeks before each trastuzumab dose; a troponin assay and NT-pro-BNP were drawn after each dose. At 3 months, LVEF remained stable at 50% in the absence of symptoms, and all biomarkers since trastuzumab initiation were within normal limits. Intervals between surveillance echocardiograms were extended to every 2 months for the remainder of trastuzumab therapy, and post-dose biomarker surveillance was discontinued. Trastuzumab therapy was then continued for 1 year without event. The patient currently remains free of recurrent cancer 2 years following the completion of trastuzumab, continues on ACE inhibitor and beta-blocker therapy, and undergoes a routine surveillance TTE annually. The most recent TTE confirms a recovery of LVEF to 60% (Video 2).

ACKNOWLEDGMENTS

JM is supported by an NIH Career Development Award (K08), Watkins Discovery Award Program and Cardiovascular Leadership Council Investigator Award (both by Brigham and Women's Hospital).

SUPPLEMENTARY DATA

Supplementary data related to this article can be found online at: http://dx.doi.org/10.1016/j.mcna.2012.07.008.

REFERENCES

1. Dahabreh IJ, Linardou H, Siannis F, et al. Trastuzumab in the adjuvant treatment of early-stage breast cancer: a systematic review and meta-analysis of randomized controlled trials. Oncologist 2008;13(6):620–30.
2. Bonadonna G, Monfardini S, De Lena M, et al. Phase I and preliminary phase II evaluation of Adriamycin (NSC 123127). Cancer Res 1970;30(10):2572–82.

3. Von Hoff DD, Rozencweig M, Layard M, et al. Daunomycin-induced cardiotoxicity in children and adults. A review of 110 cases. Am J Med 1977;62(2):200–8.
4. Wojnowski L, Kulle B, Schirmer M, et al. NAD(P)H oxidase and multidrug resistance protein genetic polymorphisms are associated with doxorubicin-induced cardiotoxicity. Circulation 2005;112(24):3754–62.
5. Tirelli U, Errante D, Van Glabbeke M, et al. CHOP is the standard regimen in patients > or = 70 years of age with intermediate-grade and high-grade non-Hodgkin's lymphoma: results of a randomized study of the European Organization for Research and Treatment of Cancer Lymphoma Cooperative Study Group. J Clin Oncol 1998;16(1):27–34.
6. Luminari S, Montanini A, Caballero D, et al. Nonpegylated liposomal doxorubicin (MyocetTM) combination (R-COMP) chemotherapy in elderly patients with diffuse large B-cell lymphoma (DLBCL): results from the phase II EUR018 trial. Ann Oncol 2010;21(7):1492–9.
7. Sawaya H, Sebag IA, Plana JC, et al. Assessment of echocardiography and biomarkers for the extended prediction of cardiotoxicity in patients treated with anthracyclines, taxanes and trastuzumab. Circ Cardiovasc Imaging 2012. [Epub ahead of print].
8. Unverferth DV, Fertel RH, Talley RL, et al. The effect of first-dose doxorubicin on the cyclic nucleotide levels of the human myocardium. Toxicol Appl Pharmacol 1981;60(1):151–4.
9. Lipshultz SE, Miller TL, Scully RE, et al. Changes in cardiac biomarkers during doxorubicin treatment of pediatric patients with high-risk acute lymphoblastic leukemia: associations with long-term echocardiographic outcomes. J Clin Oncol 2012;30(10):1042–9.
10. Smith LA, Cornelius VR, Plummer CJ, et al. Cardiotoxicity of anthracycline agents for the treatment of cancer: systematic review and meta-analysis of randomised controlled trials. BMC Cancer 2010;10:337.
11. Von Hoff DD, Layard MW, Basa P, et al. Risk factors for doxorubicin-induced congestive heart failure. Ann Intern Med 1979;91(5):710–7.
12. Lipshultz SE, Colan SD, Gelber RD, et al. Late cardiac effects of doxorubicin therapy for acute lymphoblastic leukemia in childhood. N Engl J Med 1991;324(12):808–15.
13. van der Pal HJ, van Dalen EC, Hauptmann M, et al. Cardiac function in 5-year survivors of childhood cancer: a long-term follow-up study. Arch Intern Med 2010;170(14):1247–55.
14. Lefrak EA, Pitha J, Rosenheim S, et al. A clinicopathologic analysis of Adriamycin cardiotoxicity. Cancer 1973;32(2):302–14.
15. Lipshultz SE, Lipsitz SR, Mone SM, et al. Female sex and drug dose as risk factors for late cardiotoxic effects of doxorubicin therapy for childhood cancer. N Engl J Med 1995;332(26):1738–43.
16. Sawyer DB, Peng X, Chen B, et al. Mechanisms of anthracycline cardiac injury: can we identify strategies for cardioprotection? Prog Cardiovasc Dis 2010;53(2):105–13.
17. Gianni L, Herman EH, Lipshultz SE, et al. Anthracycline cardiotoxicity: from bench to bedside. J Clin Oncol 2008;26(22):3777–84.
18. Lipshultz SE, Scully RE, Lipsitz SR, et al. Assessment of dexrazoxane as a cardioprotectant in doxorubicin-treated children with high-risk acute lymphoblastic leukaemia: long-term follow-up of a prospective, randomised, multicentre trial. Lancet Oncol 2010;11(10):950–61.
19. Lipshultz SE, Rifai N, Dalton VM, et al. The effect of dexrazoxane on myocardial injury in doxorubicin-treated children with acute lymphoblastic leukemia. N Engl J Med 2004;351(2):145–53.

20. Fuller SJ, Sivarajah K, Sugden PH. ErbB receptors, their ligands, and the consequences of their activation and inhibition in the myocardium. J Mol Cell Cardiol 2008;44(5):831–54.

21. Hynes NE, Lane HA. ERBB receptors and cancer: the complexity of targeted inhibitors. Nat Rev Cancer 2005;5(5):341–54.

22. Slamon DJ, Leyland-Jones B, Shak S, et al. Use of chemotherapy plus a monoclonal antibody against HER2 for metastatic breast cancer that overexpresses HER2. N Engl J Med 2001;344(11):783–92.

23. Nabholtz JM, Reese DM, Lindsay MA, et al. HER2-positive breast cancer: update on Breast Cancer International Research Group trials. Clin Breast Cancer 2002; 3(Suppl 2):S75–9.

24. Nakamura S, Ando M, Masuda N, et al. Randomized phase II study of primary systemic chemotherapy and trastuzumab for operable HER2 positive breast cancer. Clin Breast Cancer 2012;12(1):49–56.

25. Borg A, Baldetorp B, Ferno M, et al. ERBB2 amplification in breast cancer with a high rate of proliferation. Oncogene 1991;6(1):137–43.

26. Slamon DJ, Clark GM, Wong SG, et al. Human breast cancer: correlation of relapse and survival with amplification of the HER-2/neu oncogene. Science 1987;235(4785):177–82.

27. Rana P, Sridhar SS. Efficacy and tolerability of lapatinib in the management of breast cancer. Breast Cancer (Auckl) 2012;6:67–77.

28. Chen MH, Kerkela R, Force T. Mechanisms of cardiac dysfunction associated with tyrosine kinase inhibitor cancer therapeutics. Circulation 2008;118(1): 84–95.

29. Geyer CE, Forster J, Lindquist D, et al. Lapatinib plus capecitabine for HER2-positive advanced breast cancer. N Engl J Med 2006;355(26):2733–43.

30. Johnston S, Pippen J Jr, Pivot X, et al. Lapatinib combined with letrozole versus letrozole and placebo as first-line therapy for postmenopausal hormone receptor-positive metastatic breast cancer. J Clin Oncol 2009;27(33):5538–46.

31. Telli ML, Hunt SA, Carlson RW, et al. Trastuzumab-related cardiotoxicity: calling into question the concept of reversibility. J Clin Oncol 2007;25(23): 3525–33.

32. Perez EA, Koehler M, Byrne J, et al. Cardiac safety of lapatinib: pooled analysis of 3689 patients enrolled in clinical trials. Mayo Clin Proc 2008;83(6):679–86.

33. Ewer MS, Lippman SM. Type II chemotherapy-related cardiac dysfunction: time to recognize a new entity. J Clin Oncol 2005;23(13):2900–2.

34. Baliga RR, Pimental DR, Zhao YY, et al. NRG-1-induced cardiomyocyte hypertrophy. Role of PI-3-kinase, p70(S6K), and MEK-MAPK-RSK. Am J Physiol 1999;277(5 Pt 2):H2026–37.

35. Kuramochi Y, Guo X, Sawyer DB. Neuregulin activates erbB2-dependent src/FAK signaling and cytoskeletal remodeling in isolated adult rat cardiac myocytes. J Mol Cell Cardiol 2006;41(2):228–35.

36. Fukazawa R, Miller TA, Kuramochi Y, et al. Neuregulin-1 protects ventricular myocytes from anthracycline-induced apoptosis via erbB4-dependent activation of PI3-kinase/Akt. J Mol Cell Cardiol 2003;35(12):1473–9.

37. De Keulenaer GW, Doggen K, Lemmens K. The vulnerability of the heart as a pluricellular paracrine organ: lessons from unexpected triggers of heart failure in targeted ErbB2 anticancer therapy. Circ Res 2010;106(1):35–46.

38. Grazette LP, Boecker W, Matsui T, et al. Inhibition of ErbB2 causes mitochondrial dysfunction in cardiomyocytes: implications for Herceptin-induced cardiomyopathy. J Am Coll Cardiol 2004;44(11):2231–8.

39. Gordon LI, Burke MA, Singh AT, et al. Blockade of the erbB2 receptor induces cardiomyocyte death through mitochondrial and reactive oxygen species-dependent pathways. J Biol Chem 2009;284(4):2080–7.
40. Imai K, Takaoka A. Comparing antibody and small-molecule therapies for cancer. Nat Rev Cancer 2006;6(9):714–27.
41. Spector NL, Yarden Y, Smith B, et al. Activation of AMP-activated protein kinase by human EGF receptor 2/EGF receptor tyrosine kinase inhibitor protects cardiac cells. Proc Natl Acad Sci U S A 2007;104(25):10607–12.
42. Nayyar S, Magalski A, Khumri TM, et al. Contrast administration reduces interobserver variability in determination of left ventricular ejection fraction in patients with left ventricular dysfunction and good baseline endocardial border delineation. Am J Cardiol 2006;98(8):1110–4.
43. Kurt M, Shaikh KA, Peterson L, et al. Impact of contrast echocardiography on evaluation of ventricular function and clinical management in a large prospective cohort. J Am Coll Cardiol 2009;53(9):802–10.
44. Schwartz RG, McKenzie WB, Alexander J, et al. Congestive heart failure and left ventricular dysfunction complicating doxorubicin therapy. Seven-year experience using serial radionuclide angiocardiography. Am J Med 1987;82(6): 1109–18.
45. Patel CD, Balakrishnan VB, Kumar L, et al. Does left ventricular diastolic function deteriorate earlier than left ventricular systolic function in anthracycline cardiotoxicity? Hell J Nucl Med 2010;13(3):233–7.
46. Di Lisi D, Bonura F, Macaione F, et al. Chemotherapy-induced cardiotoxicity: role of the conventional echocardiography and the tissue Doppler. Minerva Cardioangiol 2011;59(4):301–8.
47. Radulescu D, Pripon S, Radulescu LI, et al. Left ventricular diastolic performance in breast cancer survivors treated with anthracyclines. Acta Cardiol 2008;63(1): 27–32.
48. Pudil R, Horacek JM, Strasova A, et al. Monitoring of the very early changes of left ventricular diastolic function in patients with acute leukemia treated with anthracyclines. Exp Oncol 2008;30(2):160–2.
49. Sawaya H, Sebag IA, Plana JC, et al. Early detection and prediction of cardiotoxicity in chemotherapy-treated patients. Am J Cardiol 2011;107(9):1375–80.
50. Al-Biltagi M, Abd Rab Elrasoul Tolba O, El-Shanshory MR, et al. Strain echocardiography in early detection of doxorubicin-induced left ventricular dysfunction in children with acute lymphoblastic leukemia. ISRN Pediatr 2012; 2012:870549.
51. Stoodley PW, Richards DA, Hui R, et al. Two-dimensional myocardial strain imaging detects changes in left ventricular systolic function immediately after anthracycline chemotherapy. Eur J Echocardiogr 2011;12(12):945–52.
52. Hare JL, Brown JK, Leano R, et al. Use of myocardial deformation imaging to detect preclinical myocardial dysfunction before conventional measures in patients undergoing breast cancer treatment with trastuzumab. Am Heart J 2009;158(2):294–301.
53. Walker J, Bhullar N, Fallah-Rad N, et al. Role of three-dimensional echocardiography in breast cancer: comparison with two-dimensional echocardiography, multiple-gated acquisition scans, and cardiac magnetic resonance imaging. J Clin Oncol 2010;28(21):3429–36.
54. Hamada H, Ohkubo T, Maeda M, et al. Evaluation of cardiac reserved function by high-dose dobutamine-stress echocardiography in asymptomatic anthracycline-treated survivors of childhood cancer. Pediatr Int 2006;48(3):313–20.

55. Lanzarini L, Bossi G, Laudisa ML, et al. Lack of clinically significant cardiac dysfunction during intermediate dobutamine doses in long-term childhood cancer survivors exposed to anthracyclines. Am Heart J 2000;140(2):315–23.

56. Sieswerda E, Kremer LC, Vidmar S, et al. Exercise echocardiography in asymptomatic survivors of childhood cancer treated with anthracyclines: a prospective follow-up study. Pediatr Blood Cancer 2010;54(4):579–84.

57. de Geus-Oei LF, Mavinkurve-Groothuis AM, Bellersen L, et al. Scintigraphic techniques for early detection of cancer treatment-induced cardiotoxicity. J Nucl Med 2011;52(4):560–71.

58. Oberholzer K, Kunz RP, Dittrich M, et al. [Anthracycline-induced cardiotoxicity: cardiac MRI after treatment for childhood cancer]. Rofo 2004;176(9):1245–50 [in German].

59. Fallah-Rad N, Lytwyn M, Fang T, et al. Delayed contrast enhancement cardiac magnetic resonance imaging in trastuzumab induced cardiomyopathy. J Cardiovasc Magn Reson 2008;10:5.

60. Douglas PS, Khandheria B, Stainback RF, et al. ACCF/ASE/ACEP/ASNC/SCAI/SCCT/SCMR 2007 appropriateness criteria for transthoracic and transesophageal echocardiography: a report of the American College of Cardiology Foundation Quality Strategic Directions Committee Appropriateness Criteria Working Group, American Society of Echocardiography, American College of Emergency Physicians, American Society of Nuclear Cardiology, Society for Cardiovascular Angiography and Interventions, Society of Cardiovascular Computed Tomography, and the Society for Cardiovascular Magnetic Resonance endorsed by the American College of Chest Physicians and the Society of Critical Care Medicine. J Am Coll Cardiol 2007;50(2):187–204.

61. Hendel RC, Berman DS, Di Carli MF, et al. ACCF/ASNC/ACR/AHA/ASE/SCCT/SCMR/SNM 2009 appropriate use criteria for cardiac radionuclide imaging: a report of the American College of Cardiology Foundation Appropriate Use Criteria Task Force, the American Society of Nuclear Cardiology, the American College of Radiology, the American Heart Association, the American Society of Echocardiography, the Society of Cardiovascular Computed Tomography, the Society for Cardiovascular Magnetic Resonance, and the Society of Nuclear Medicine. Circulation 2009;119(22):e561–87.

62. Hendel RC, Patel MR, Kramer CM, et al. ACCF/ACR/SCCT/SCMR/ASNC/NASCI/SCAI/SIR 2006 appropriateness criteria for cardiac computed tomography and cardiac magnetic resonance imaging: a report of the American College of Cardiology Foundation Quality Strategic Directions Committee Appropriateness Criteria Working Group, American College of Radiology, Society of Cardiovascular Computed Tomography, Society for Cardiovascular Magnetic Resonance, American Society of Nuclear Cardiology, North American Society for Cardiac Imaging, Society for Cardiovascular Angiography and Interventions, and Society of Interventional Radiology. J Am Coll Cardiol 2006;48(7):1475–97.

63. Cardinale D, Sandri MT, Martinoni A, et al. Left ventricular dysfunction predicted by early troponin I release after high-dose chemotherapy. J Am Coll Cardiol 2000;36(2):517–22.

64. Cardinale D, Sandri MT, Martinoni A, et al. Myocardial injury revealed by plasma troponin I in breast cancer treated with high-dose chemotherapy. Ann Oncol 2002;13(5):710–5.

65. Cardinale D, Sandri MT, Colombo A, et al. Prognostic value of troponin I in cardiac risk stratification of cancer patients undergoing high-dose chemotherapy. Circulation 2004;109(22):2749–54.

66. Sandri MT, Salvatici M, Cardinale D, et al. N-terminal pro-B-type natriuretic peptide after high-dose chemotherapy: a marker predictive of cardiac dysfunction? Clin Chem 2005;51(8):1405–10.

67. Cochet A, Quilichini G, Dygai-Cochet I, et al. Baseline diastolic dysfunction as a predictive factor of trastuzumab-mediated cardiotoxicity after adjuvant anthracycline therapy in breast cancer. Breast Cancer Res Treat 2011;130(3): 845–54.

68. Fallah-Rad N, Walker JR, Wassef A, et al. The utility of cardiac biomarkers, tissue velocity and strain imaging, and cardiac magnetic resonance imaging in predicting early left ventricular dysfunction in patients with human epidermal growth factor receptor II-positive breast cancer treated with adjuvant trastuzumab therapy. J Am Coll Cardiol 2011;57(22):2263–70.

69. Schmitz KH, Prosnitz RG, Schwartz AL, et al. Prospective surveillance and management of cardiac toxicity and health in breast cancer survivors. Cancer 2012;118(Suppl 8):2270–6.

70. Aapro M, Bernard-Marty C, Brain EG, et al. Anthracycline cardiotoxicity in the elderly cancer patient: a SIOG expert position paper. Ann Oncol 2011;22(2): 257–67.

71. Hunt SA, Abraham WT, Chin MH, et al. 2009 Focused update incorporated into the ACC/AHA 2005 guidelines for the diagnosis and management of heart failure in adults a report of the American College of Cardiology Foundation/American Heart Association Task Force on Practice Guidelines developed in collaboration with the International Society for Heart and Lung Transplantation. J Am Coll Cardiol 2009;53(15):e1–90.

72. Cardinale D, Colombo A, Lamantia G, et al. Anthracycline-induced cardiomyopathy: clinical relevance and response to pharmacologic therapy. J Am Coll Cardiol 2010;55(3):213–20.

73. Lu CY, Srasuebkul P, Drew AK, et al. Positive spillover effects of prescribing requirements: increased cardiac testing in patients treated with trastuzumab for HER2+ metastatic breast cancer. Intern Med J 2011. [Epub ahead of print].

74. Bellenger NG, Burgess MI, Ray SG, et al. Comparison of left ventricular ejection fraction and volumes in heart failure by echocardiography, radionuclide ventriculography and cardiovascular magnetic resonance; are they interchangeable? Eur Heart J 2000;21(16):1387–96.

75. Verma S, Ewer MS. Is cardiotoxicity being adequately assessed in current trials of cytotoxic and targeted agents in breast cancer? Ann Oncol 2011;22(5):1011–8.

Index

Note: Page numbers of article titles are in **boldface** type.

A

A Placebo-Controlled, Double Blind, Parallel Arm Trial to Assess the Efficacy of Dronedarone 400 Bid for the Prevention of Cardiovascular Hospitalization or Death from Any Cause in Patients With Atrial Fibrillation/Atrial Flutter (ATHENA), 993

A Trial of Omecamtiv Mecarbil to Increase Contractility in Acute Heart Failure (ATOMIC-AHF), 949

N-Acetyl-β-D-glucosaminidase, as biomarker, 966

ACTIVE (Atrial Fibrillation Clopidogrel Trial with Irbsartan for Prevention of Vascular Events) trial, 995–996

Acute Infarction Ramipril Efficiency (AIRE), 919

Acute Study of Clinical Effectiveness of Nesiritide in Decompensated Heart Failure (ASCEND-HF), 945

Adipositas cordis, 980

AF-CHR (Atrial Fibrillation in Congestive Heart Failure) trial, 990–991

African-American Heart Failure Trial, 928–929

AIRE (Acute Infarction Ramipril Efficiency), 919

Albuminuria, as biomarker, 966

Aldosterone, in heart failure, 884–885, 894

Aldosterone antagonists, 897–898, 920, 924–925

Amiodarone, for atrial fibrillation, 990

ANDROMEDA (Antiarrhythmic Trial with Dronedarone in Moderate to Severe CHF Evaluation Morbidity Decrease), 993

Anemia, 979–980

Angioedema, from angiotensin-converting enzyme inhibitors, 923

Angiotensin, in heart failure, 884–885, 894

Angiotensin receptor blockers, 897–898, 920, 923–924, 995

Angiotensin-converting enzyme, in heart failure, 884–885

Angiotensin-converting enzyme inhibitors, 884–885, 898, 918–923, 963

  adverse effects of, 921–923

  dosage of, 919–921

  for atrial fibrillation, 995

  in diabetes, 977

  safety of, 921–923

  trials of, 918–919

Anthracyclines, cardiomyopathy due to, 1003–1005

Antiarrhythmic Trial with Dronedarone in Moderate to Severe CHF Evaluation Morbidity Decrease (ANDROMEDA), 993

Antiplatelet therapy, for atrial fibrillation, 996

Antithrombosis therapy, for atrial fibrillation, 995–996

Apnea, sleep, 979

ASCEND-HF (Acute Study of Clinical Effectiveness of Nesiritide in Decompensated Heart Failure), 945

Med Clin N Am 96 (2012) 1021–1031

http://dx.doi.org/10.1016/S0025-7125(12)00143-5

0025-7125/12/$ – see front matter © 2012 Elsevier Inc. All rights reserved.

medical.theclinics.com

Metabolism
Fast and Free Publication

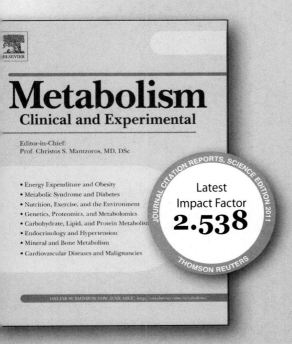

Editor-in-Chief:
Christos S. Mantzoros,
MD, DSc

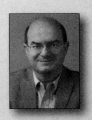

Associate Editors:
Catherine M. Gordon
Young-Bum Kim
Jonathan Williams

Metabolism publishes high-quality original research related to all aspects of human metabolism. Papers in any aspect of translational and clinical metabolic research will be considered for publication including:

- Energy Expenditure and Obesity
- Metabolic Syndrome and Diabetes
- Nutrition, Exercise, and the Environment
- Genetics, Proteomics, and Metabolomics
- Carbohydrate, Lipid, and Protein Metabolism
- Endocrinology and Hypertension
- Mineral and Bone Metabolism
- Cardiovascular Diseases and Malignancies

Why Submit to Metabolism?

Online submission and peer review at
http://ees.elsevier.com/metabolism/
Fast, high-quality editorial process
No page charges
Eminent editorial advisory board
Global readership
Impact Factor is 2.538*
12 issues per year

Journal Citation Reports, published by Thomson Reuters, 2011

Submit now!
You can submit online
and find out more at
http://ees.elsevier.com/metabolism

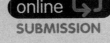

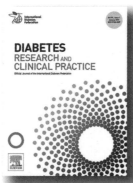
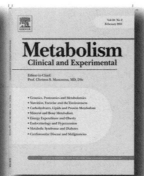
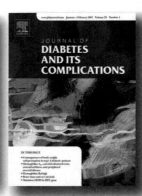
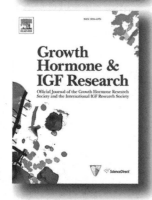
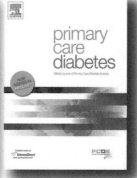
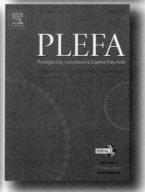

Moving?

Make sure your subscription moves with you!

To notify us of your new address, find your **Clinics Account Number** (located on your mailing label above your name), and contact customer service at:

Email: journalscustomerservice-usa@elsevier.com

800-654-2452 (subscribers in the U.S. & Canada)
314-447-8871 (subscribers outside of the U.S. & Canada)

Fax number: 314-447-8029

Elsevier Health Sciences Division
Subscription Customer Service
3251 Riverport Lane
Maryland Heights, MO 63043

*To ensure uninterrupted delivery of your subscription, please notify us at least 4 weeks in advance of move.

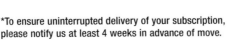